Computer Aid in Gastroenterology

Frontiers of Gastrointestinal Research

Vol. 7

Series Editor

P. Rozen, Tel Aviv

KARGER

S. Karger · Basel · München · Paris · London · New York · Tokyo · Sydney

Computer Aid in Gastroenterology

Volume Editors
P. Rozen, Tel Aviv
F.T. de Dombal, Leeds

37 figures and 39 tables, 1984

KARGER

S. Karger · Basel · München · Paris · London · New York · Tokyo · Sydney

Frontiers of Gastrointestinal Research

National Library of Medicine, Cataloging in Publication
Computer aid in gastroenterology
Volume editors, P. Rozen, F.T. de Dombal. – Basel; New York: Karger, 1984. –
(Frontiers of gastrointestinal research; v. 7)
Includes index.
1. Computers 2. Gastroenterology I. De Dombal, F.T. II. Rozen, P. (Paul) III. Series
W1 FR946E v. 7 [WI 26.5 C738]
ISBN 3–8055–3770–0

Drug Dosage

The authors and the publisher have exerted every effort to ensure that drug selection and dosage set forth in this text are in accord with current recommendations and practice at the time of publication. However, in view of ongoing research, changes in government regulations, and the constant flow of information relating to drug therapy and drug reactions, the reader is urged to check the package insert for each drug for any change in indications and dosage and for added warnings and precautions. This is particularly important when the recommended agent is a new and/or infrequently employed drug.

Satz: Satzstudio Frohberg, D-6463 Freigericht
Printed in Switzerland by Thür AG Offsetdruck, Pratteln
ISBN 3–8055–3770–0

Contents

Introduction

Why have gastroenterologists not gone out and bought computers the way they have endoscopes? Physicians usually love technology, and gastroenterologists are among the most ardent. Abandoning their once beloved X-ray machines, they have thrust the new endoscopes into every available orifice so fervently that over the past decade or so gastroenterology has moved from a person-oriented to a disease-oriented specialty. To a large extent, I am sorry about that, because it has always seemed to me that the gastroenterologist should not regard himself or herself simply as an endoscopist, the force which propells the instrument, but he or she should recognize it as simply a useful tool, one which should remain our servant and not our substitute. Yet ask any gastrointestinal resident what he wants in a training program, and he will usually tell you that he wants the opportunity to perform as many endoscopies as possible. He does not even mention learning how to use a computer. To a large extent, I fear that young men and women who go into gastroenterology today are inherently prehensile, the endoscope an extension of their hands. They do not seem to recognize that the computer, on the other hand, is an extension of their minds. Most gastroenterologists are more enthusiastic about what they can see in the patient than about what they can hear from him.

Why then has there not been the same explosion of interest in computers as there has been in ultrasound or computed tomography or endoscopy? The third-party payers do not pay for the use of a computer, and while the access to information from the computer could be as valuable, or even more valuable, than that from the endoscope, physicians in training and in practice have little stimulus to learn about computers because to gain acces costs money. That is not the major reason, however. The real reason, I suspect, is that my generation of physicians are still afraid that the computer will 'take over'. We fear that it will run off with our practice and that our hard-won expertise can be quickly duplicated by a kind of robot. Tireless servants, computers have such magnificent memories, can search the literature quicker than we can and can even do it at night. The old science fiction notions of the magnificent machines running the cities for the benefit of the citizens who atrophy into parasites and sybarites with nothing to do but enjoy themselves lurk in the back of our minds. We really do fear that the computer will become the physicians and we the *dieners* of the machine.

Clearly, so far people prefer to be taken care of by other people, but computers have now arrived at the stage at which physicians generally should begin to learn how to take them into more active partnership and not wait until they are forced to do so. I like to look at the computer as working for me. The word processor shortens the time to revise a manuscript, carries programs to make files and indices much more available and, in the latest software, makes it possible to compile bibliographies, to rearrange them and renumber them, and to gain access to other bibliographic programs. The *modem* in my friend's office gives her access to MEDLINE and to much more in the Yale mainframe computer at a trifling cost. More important for the clinician, the computer can jog his memory and, with programs appropriately developing, can even suggest what the diagnosis ought to be. All this is done tactfully, even for a machine. In the office, computers arranging clinical data, so that it can be quickly analyzed, should be able to tell a physician what his experience has been with drug X for disease Y and how that compares with what the literature says. And much more!

Yet, despite all of these current common miracles and more to come, most physicians remain sadly computer illiterate. That will not be true of the generation now in grammar school. My wife teaches science and computers to schoolchildren in New Haven and tells me how remarkably children as young as 5 or 6 years take to playing with computers and how their elders – of 8 or 9 years can do things with computers that they cannot even explain to their teacher. Somehow they have 'cathexed' the computer. Clearly, anyone who has watched college students working with computers will recognize that they are as comfortable with computers as their parents were with typewriters and that a need for a book such as the one you are now reading will quickly pass. Yet for now, it is extremely important, particularly for the generation over 30 which encompasses most practicing and academic physicians. For most of us, the computer remains something of a mystery, a challenge, an enigma, and – let us say it – a danger. Most of us do not trust computers very much despite all that I have just said. After reading this book, I realize that I must know them much better than I do and that this book has helped me to an awareness of their enormous potential.

What Drs. *Rozen* and *de Dombal* have tried to do then is to set out a primer and a training manual for the gastroenterologist. Equally important, they have provided an extensive bibliography, so that you can learn even more by reading the relevant literature. I have benefitted enormously from reading this book, and I will return to my office and library with renewed enthusiasm for the future in the belief that, if my memory fails, the computer will give me renewed rigor. I am grateful to them.

Howard M. Spiro, MD, Yale University School of Medicine, Box 3333,
333 Cedar Street, New Haven, CT 06510 (USA)

Front. gastrointest. Res., vol. 7, pp. 1–13 (Karger, Basel 1984)

Computer Aid in Gastroenterology: An Overview

P. Rozen

Municipal Governmental Medical Center and Sackler School of Medicine, Tel Aviv, Israel

During a review of the subject of computer assistance in gastroenterology [51], the impression was that of a paucity of germane literature. However, since 1980, there has been an increasing number of publications on the use of computers in fields relevant to gastroenterology (GI), but still prominent is the lack of interest of most gastroenterologists and GI journals. This apparently is changing, as can be seen by the holding of special sessions on the subject in The World Congress of Gastroenterology, Stockholm 1982; the XIXth International SMIER Congress (Société Médicale Internationale d'Endoscopie et de Radiocinéma), Nancy 1983; the American College of Gastroenterology Meeting, Boston 1983; and Digestive Disease Week, Washington 1983.

This chapter will address itself to recent, relevant publications of general and specific interest to gastroenterologists.

Computer Literature of General Interest

It would be valuable to start with the review by *Friedman and Gustafson* [17] in 1977, on computers in clinical medicine. They pointed out the faults of the hardware and software available, making the then-existing computer system uncomfortable for physicians to use, time-consuming and often not effective. To some extent, as pointed out by *Llaurado* [36] in 1982, the rapid development of microprocessors has solved the hardware problem, especially costs. However, software high level languages, such as FORTRAN are inadequate for everyday needs. The continuous and rapid changes in medical practise require time-consuming and therefore expensive programming. While improved languages, such as PASCAL or MUMPS, are rarely used or available commercially and therefore not well known.

As *Diamond* [12] pointed out, we must accept the computer as a partner where the physician has the last word. This is made easier with the advent of the personal computer which, as found by *Gorry* [23] is more compatible with the individual physician. *Anderson and Jay* [1] analysed the difficulties in getting physicians to utilize existing computer services. They demonstrated that the best approach is two-step, first getting the key influential staff members to be involved, and then their example will carry the remaining staff with them.

As stated, very little has been done about computerizing GI services. We can learn from the examples of radiology departments [4, 32] whose organizational structure is not dissimilar to that of GI; namely scheduling, equipment care, reports and billing, etc.

Health Questionnaires

These have been used in several screening centers, as printed cards for off-line computer entry, optical forms or punch cards, but without clear mass acceptance [51]. *Trell* et al. [58, 59] have successfully used a fully interactive system in a multiphasic preventive health program in Sweden. This is based on a minicomputer with special simplified keyboards for data entry. It requires a degree of patient sophistication and sometimes the old-fashioned off-line forms are used. In addition, the nursing staff enter the results of laboratory tests directly into the computer in order to save time and information loss. Their experience with 15,000 examinations over 3 years is favorable.

Medical Records

The computer recording, storage and analysis of medical information requires the use of standardized language. This is well reviewed by *Côté and Robboy* [7], in 1980. They describe the WHO International Classification of Disease (ICD); the need for a more flexible hierarchical system led to SNOP, the Systematized Nomenclature of Pathology. This in turn has been further extended to SNOMED which is a comprehensive multiaxial nomenclature for the entire health care system. It is computer compatible and its logical open-ended modules allow future extensions. As *Côté and Robboy* [7] point out, and from personal experience, this all-encompassing system is too voluminous to be easily handled, and abbreviated versions should be made available. An example of its use is given in this volume by *Jeanty*.

Various medical schools have been in the forefront of developing information systems for computerizing medical records for storage, retrieval, analysis and ultimately to act as a data bank for future patient management based on past experience. Notable have been the contributions from the Stanford Medical Center [18, 62], where they developed computer-compatible, structured forms for use as the patient's chart. This is obviously an off-line system which allowed them to develop an extensive data bank. Similar projects have been performed at Duke University cardiac unit [49] and they pointed out that success required the active integration of biostatisticians, computer scientists, bioengineers, epidemiologists and clinicians. This is best performed by having them work together *in the clinical unit*. In 1975, the Massachusetts General Hospital Laboratory of Computer Science developed a computer-stored ambulatory record system (COSTAR) and medical query language (MQL) based on MUMPS (Massachusetts General Hospital Utility Multiprogramming System). The record system, like most others described, is based on physician-recorded worksheets ready for technician computer entry. What is important is their use of a specialized, sophisticated, high-level language which unfortunately is not yet popular commercially. The real-time handling of clinical data is described by *Huet* et al. [27] at the University of Paris intensive care unit. Using a microcomputer they developed an on-line dictionary of 2,700 key words commonly used by their physicians. This allows for direct data entry by secretary and physician, and analysis and printing of medical records.

The need for a general purpose data base management system for developing and changing needs in both hospital information systems and clinical research was emphasized by *Lustman* [37] who described a new model to answer this problem. *Baker and Shaffer* [2] from the UK, described in 1982, a package for processing patient questionnaire text and data, preparing them for statistical analysis. In 1979, *Fox* [16] reviewed the overall hospital needs for computing services in the UK. He addressed the human problem of computer acceptance and recommended, as we have found, that it is best to start with small, dedicated minicomputers to satisfy local needs and then subsequently integrate them into a network and the centralized hospital system. Hospital information systems (HIS) are becoming increasingly important. *Hadidi* et al. [24] emphasized the importance of clearly defining and evaluating candidate components for automation, based on first identifying the most influential hospital staff and then obtaining their recommendations! More on the HIS is given in the chapter by *Lichtenstein*.

In general, the overall impression is of a confusing array of incompatible programs for data management. Somehow, we must standardize and develop compatible and expandible programs for online medical data management.

Pathology Reporting and Image Analysis

Recently, there have been many reports of the successful utilization of computer technology for data management and image analysis in pathology. These experiences are eminently applicable to GI.

MacDonald et al. [38] described the use of a simple cheap system for a small-to-medium-sized department, based on preformated report forms, standardized terminology and a microcomputer, while *Davey and Vaughan* [10] used mark sense cards for each major body system or area of surgical pathology. These are processed by a card reader and resulted in a reduction of clerical time and the generation of concise reports. A more sophisticated approach was described by *Robboy* et al. [48] and *Foster* et al. [15] from Boston, using on-line data entry, SNOMED terminology and MUMPS programming. This allows data entry, storage, retrieval, report preparation, analysis, billing and more! The most difficult part for the secretarial service to manage is the coding. This is done by hand and can lead to inaccuracies. Another problem, that of integrating the pathology services of 5 hospitals, was well described by *Cechner* [5] in Cleveland. The analysis of the hardware problems resulted in the successful set-up of a network of micro- and minicomputers.

As pointed out by *Hoshino* [26] from Kyoto, computerization is inevitable for cytological pattern recognition for basic and clinical cell biology studies; while *Zajicek* et al. [64] from Jerusalem described automated image processing of the colon crypt epithelium, which could be useful for standardized experimental studies. A further extension of computer image analysis has been by the electron microscopists [53]. Till recently, they required large computers and generated poor quality images, newer hardware and software developments have reversed the situation.

References

Searching for references is usually done by hand, based on memory and the Index Medicus. A more expensive, but occasionally incomplete search, can be performed via reference banks such as MEDLINE. For those who wish to generate their own data base of references on a microcomputer, programs are available to facilitate this. Paperbase, Wight Scientific

UK, and Sci-Mate, ISI Philadelphia [21, 22], will allow the storage and manipulation of references. It should be remembered that the microcomputer has limited storage, for this reason the ISI program is advantageous. The microcomputer can be connected by phone line, via a modum, to the ISI data banks. Note that somebody still has to enter and update the references, no small task! Having Current Contents® on-line will facilitate this. This aspect of computer application is further addressed by *Bernstein* and co-workers in another chapter.

Software Catalog

Is available from the publishers Elsevier, the Netherlands, listing twice yearly international software for micro- and minicomputers. Not specifically for medical fields.

Computer Aid in Decision Making

Using a computer to assist in making a diagnosis, recommending further tests or therapy, has been the ultimate goal of many workers impressed by the computers ability to store and analyse information and provide a rapid response. This is apparently possible and practical for well-defined processes (see chapters by *Clamp* and co-workers and *de Dombal*) but runs into difficulties with complex and multiple medical problems. The difficulty being an inability to transfer to the computer the logic process used by the *experienced* physician to reach a decision. An analysis and understanding of the thinking process is therefore critical, in order to transfer it to computer logic. This had been looked at by *Pauker and Kassirer* [44] using a decision tree model. This is suitable when considering a single disease, where decisions can be based on the logical, statistical estimates of the probable value of alternatives for diagnostic procedures, therapy, etc. This model is eminently computer adaptable and the same authors [45] have prepared programs for personal computers that are within the ability and financial range of clinical practice. The criticism of this system is that to some extent it is subjective, requiring the physician's estimates of probability. Whereas a large computer data bank of past experience would be more objective and, hopefully, accurate.

Using another approach, the psychological process used to solve complex diagnostic problems, such as a clinicopathological exercise, has been analyzed by *Eddy and Clanton* [13]. They pointed out that the size and complexity of the problem will often make it impossible to mentally manipulate all the probabilities, and so the Bayes' theorem is not useful in such a case.

They suggested using a heuristic model; firstly, the problem is reduced in size by aggregating the findings, then choosing a 'pivot' or pathognomonic finding and generating a list of probable causes; the list is then pruned, a diagnosis selected and finally validated. This approach has been used in developing Internists–I, an experimental computer-based diagnostic consultant for internal medicine [42]. Its capabilities are based on an extensive knowledge base and the use of heuristic computer programs to construct and resolve differential diagnoses. This major project attempts to model the behavior of physicians, using heuristic principles, such as diagnosis by exlusion. The data base is organized by listing diseases in blocks, organized in a hierarchy form, from general to specific. However, the user is still required to enter his judgement on evoking strength and frequency of each clinical variable. The system is incomplete, and as the authors *Miller* et al. [42] and *Barnett* [3] point out, still cannot fully handle a complex multisystem problem as well as a specialist. This has led to the development of CADUCEUS, which is claimed to be able to manage a broad overview of clinical problems.

The systems available for computer-assisted medical decision making have been well reviewed recently [47, 63, 66] and they should be read by the uninitiated in the order of ascending complexity. *Young* [63] points out the necessity of having a large updated data base of relevant information suggesting lines of action, but showing the user the basis of its suggestions and allowing him the final choice. Computer decision support systems available are usually for clearly defined topics such as CARE, for surgical decisions; MYCIN for prescribing antibiotics; HOIS for junior house staff; and others already referred to.

Not surprisingly, it has become apparent that we must also take into account the patients' preferences in deciding between alternative means of investigation and therapy [14, 41]. So behavioral analysis, risks, gains, etc., will also have to be considered in our computer models! A good case for the importance of computer guidelines, or at least second opinions for surgical decisions, has been demonstrated by *Vayda* et al. [61] in analysing physicians' replies to hypothetical cases for surgical therapy. There were substantial differences of opinion between specialities and among the surgeons themselves!

From reviewing the literature, it would seem that at present computer systems are most useful as aids for analyzing *clearly* defined problems. More complex analyses are not well handled as yet, because of our inability to transfer our mental analytical processes to computer computations (maybe we should try the reverse?). In addition, there is at present a half-hearted physician acceptance of the role of computer technology in medicine, partly due to a lack of sophistication on our part. This will clearly change in time.

Computer Literature Related to GI

Nutrition

Parenteral nutrition is a complex subject requiring individualization and careful calculations. This lends itself to computerization [56].

Analysis of GI Symptom Complexes

Dyspepsia is a general term, referring to persistent upper GI discomfort. *Crean* et al. [8] have used computer technology to analyze and guide them in its investigation. Using a structured questionnaire, a self-administered questionnaire, endoscopy and radiology report, they obtain over 200 items of information from each patient. Their experience with 1,000 patients has provided a substantial data base. Lately, they have been using successfully, computer interrogation in place of physician interviewing. As many patients have more than one cause for their symptoms, which may be interdependent, the Bayes' theorem is not used for the symptom analysis. Each symptom is given a score, estimated from the data base, and the total score is transformed by the computer into a probability. This can then lead to management decisions regarding further tests and treatment. In their experience, such a program in Primary Health Centers, would substantially reduce hospital referrals for this symptom complex.

Esophagus

Esophageal manometry, like electrocardiography, lends itself to computer analysis. This has been used to characterize the ideal manometric techniques needed to obtain accurate recordings [43] and perform on-line analysis [60]. The hardware needed for this latter feature, similar to that used in cardiac catheterization laboratories, is unfortunately too expensive for most GI units. It analyzes the swallow, peristalsis, LES pressure and pH recordings over 24 h. These inputs are continuously transferred via a digital converter, to a microcomputer. A simpler portable system for continuous pH monitoring, with computer data analysis, is useful for the diagnosis of reflux disease [46].

Stomach

As in the esophagus, similar technology has been used for the continuous digital and analogue recording and analysis of simultaneous gastric and duodenal pH [40]. While *Laurent* [34], briefly describes his use of a microcomputer for analyzing perendoscopic measurements of gastric pH in various diseases and areas of the stomach.

Small and Large Bowel

Lengthy studies of intestinal myoelectric activity require complex and tedious analyses. Both *Summers* et al. [55] and *Crenner* et al. [9] have used computerized analytical techniques. Spike activity detected by electrodes, in dogs, in transfered via an analog-to-digital converter to a minicomputer for recording and on-line analysis.

A software package for studying drug absorption has been prepared by and is available from CIBA-Geigy (6), for use on a microcomputer. This package, which includes graphics, allows for pharmacokinetic studies of drugs following oral ingestion.

GI Tumors

In a high-incidence country, China, the computer-aided diagnosis of gastric cancer, based on a data bank of 35,500 cases, was found to be superior to X-ray or experienced physician diagnosis [65]. Whether this program can be adapted to the occident remains to be proven.

Gage [20] suggested applying threshold analysis in deciding on screening colonoscopy or colectomy to prevent cancer in colitis, and described his model. *Macrae and Williams* [39] have established a computer file for the follow-up and cancer risk assessment of patients with colorectal polyps. Using computer technology and multivariate analysis of the Erlangen registry of 2,071 colon polyps [25], the size and shape and histological types were confirmed to be important markers of potential malignancy.

Pancreas-Liver

Shichiri et al. [54], from Osaka, have developed an experimental, miniaturized, artificial endocrine pancreas. This closed loop system is based on a needle-type glucose sensor, computer calculated insulin infusing rate and pump for subcutaneous infusion. This system might initiate a new approach for the care of insulin-dependent diabetics.

Jagoe et al. [30] have developed an interactive computer method for measuring nuclear size and shape in normal livers and hepatomas. This allows for a good, objective discrimination between malignant and benign nuclei and may act as a model for other tissues.

Physicians commonly order multiple tests, especially when liver disease is suspected. They then mentally have to analyze each result separately, to exclude spurious values, and then group them and decide if the pattern formed is diagnostic of a type of liver disease. *Ryback* et al. [52] have used sophisticated statistical software, on microcomputer, to discriminate between types of liver disease, namely alcoholic from nonalcoholic. As heterogeneity, rather than homogeneity is the common finding with medical data, they have used quadratic discriminant analysis with superior results than those obtained with the usual linear discriminant analysis of pattern recognition. Another, but simpler approach to the same problem, was used by *Itoshima* et al. [28, 29] using 12 liver tests to discriminate between 8 parenchymal diseases. Based on a data bank of prior experience they gave each test a diagnostic score value and prepared a table for hand calculation [28], their first likelihood diagnosis was correct in only 50%.

They then used a microcomputer to rank the tests in order of their diagnostic value and found that eliminating 5 did not effect the diagnostic accuracy of the remaining tests [29]. Even so, their discriminative ability seems inadequate. *Lindberg* et al. [35], in Stockholm, are aiming at the computer-aided diagnosis of jaundice. To reach this goal they have followed the clinical, diagnostic and therapeutic course of 144 consecutive jaundiced patients. The analysis of the diagnostic strategies used, and experiences gained, will become the basis for choosing the optimal computer-aided approach to this clinical problem. Correctly, they make the observation that a great deal of expensive time is wasted in hospital for observation and waiting for investigations. Computer aid might hasten the diagnostic process. Similarly, *Richter* et al. [50] are utilizing decision analysis and computer modeling for the selection of accurate and efficient strategies for the diagnosis of suspected extrahepatic jaundice.

Endoscopy

The use of computer storage and analysis of endoscopy findings is dealt with in detail in another chapter. Briefly, there are reports of off-line punch card systems [19] and on-line microcomputer systems [11, 31, 33, 57]. Two commercially available systems are MicroMed, Medical Systems Ltd., UK, for use on a Sirius microcomputer with hard disc, and GI 2000, E. Levy Ltd., Tel-Aviv for an IBM or Digital, mini or personal computer.

In conclusion, there is a paucity of publications regarding the application of computer technology to GI. We are lagging behind other areas of medicine in spite of being a 'high-technology' subspecialty, possibly because of our preoccupation till now with the technical aspects. Only recently have our GI societies become aware of the topic, but still not giving it the emphasis due. Also, the key GI journals have not given prominence to the possible uses of computer technology in gastroenterology. We hope that this book will be a suitable *introduction* to the subject for the clinical gastroenterologist and thank the chapter authors for their contributions and the publishers for their patience!

References

1 Anderson, J.G.; Jay, S.J.: Utilization of computers in clinical practice - role of physician networks: preliminary communication. J. R. Soc. Med. *76*: 45–52 (1983).

2 Baker, R.D.; Shaffer, J.L.: QUEST – A package for processing questionnaire text and data. Comput. Biol. Med. *12*: 309–318 (1982).

3 Barnett, G.O.: The computer and clinical judgment. New Engl. J. Med. *307*: 493–494 (1982).

4 Barnhard, H.J.; Lane, G.B.: The computerized diagnostic radiology department: update 1982. Radiology *145*: 551–558 (1982).

5 Cechner, R.L.: A multifunction network of computers in a large pathology department. Integration of word processing, data base management, and general purpose computing using network principles. Am. J. clin. Path. *79*: 472–480 (1983).

6 Chan, K.K.H.; Wnuck, K.: Microcomputer based pharmokinetic programs for calculating absorption rate. Comput. Progr. Biomed. *16*: 27–34 (1983).

7 Côté, R.A.; Robboy, S.: Progress in medical information management. Standardized nomenclature of medicine (SNOMED). J. Am. med. Ass. *243*: 756–762 (1980).

8 Crean, G.P.; Card, W.J.; Beattie, A.D.; Holden, R.J.; James, W.B.; Knill-Jones, R.P.; Lucas, R.W.: Spiegelhalter, D.: Ulcer-like dyspepsia. Scand. J. Gastroent. *17*: suppl. 79, pp. 9–15 (1982).

9 Crenner, F.; Lambert, A.; Angel, F.; Schang, J.C.; Grenier, J.F.: Analogue automated analysis of small intestinal electromyogram. Med. biol. Eng. Comp. *20*: 151–158 (1982).

10 Davey, P.W.; Vaughan, K.D.: Computer-assisted diagnostic surgical pathology reporting. Am. J. clin. Path. *78*: 337–341 (1982).

11 Deltenre, M.; De Reuck, M.; Hermanus, A.; De Vos, A.; Burette, A.; Van Gossum, M.: Micro-computer for filing, endoscopy reports. First results. Acta endosc. *13*: 37–45 (1983).

12 Diamond, G.A.: Computer diagnosis: revolution or revelation? Int. J. Cardiol. *2*: 219–220 (1982).

13 Eddy, D.M.; Clanton, C.H.: The art of diagnosis. Solving the clinicopathological exercise. New Engl. J. Med. *306*: 1263–1268 (1982).

14 Eraker, S.A.; Politser, P.: How decisions are reached: physician and patient. Ann. intern. Med. *97*: 262–268 (1982).
15 Foster, E.A.; Stein, A.; Liberman, D.; Cooper, C.; Wolfe, H.J.: A computer-assisted surgical pathology system. Am. J. clin. Path. *78*: 328–336 (1982).
16 Fox, J.: Development of hospital computing. J. R. Soc. Med. *72*: 425–431 (1979).
17 Friedman, R.B.; Gustafson, D.H.: Computers in clinical medicine, a critical review. Comput. Biomed. Res. *10*: 199–204 (1977).
18 Fries, J.F.: A data bank for the clinician? New Engl. J. Med. *294*: 1400–1402 (1976).
19 Frühmorgen, P.: Documentation of endoscopic findings; in Frühmorgen, Classen, Endoscopy and biopsy in gastroenterology. Technique and indications, pp. 24–34 (Springer, New York 1980).
20 Gage, T.P.: Screening colonoscopy or colectomy to prevent cancer in colitis? A decision-analytic approach (Abstract). Gastroenterology *82*: 1062 (1982).
21 Garfield, E.: Introducing Sci-Mate – a menu-driven microcomputer software package for online and offline information retrieval. I. The Sci-Mate personal data manager. Current Contents *12*: 5–12 (1983).
22 Garfield, E.: Introducing Sci-Mate – a menu-driven microcomputer software package for online and offline information retrieval. II. The Sci-Mate universal online searcher. Current Contents *14*: 5–15 (1983).
23 Gorry, G.A.: The personal computer and clinical practice. Archs intern. Med. *141*: 1745–1746 (1981).
24 Hadidi, R.; Leonard, M.S.; Ashton, W.B.: A quantitative method for the selection of hospital information systems components. Comput. Biomed. Res. *15*: 250–261 (1982).
25 Hermanek, P.; Frühmorgen, P.; Guggenmoos-Holzmann, I.; Altendorf, A.; Matek, W.: The malignant potential of colorectal polyps. A new statistical approach. Endoscopy *15*: 16–20 (1983).
26 Hoshino, K.: How useful are microcomputers in histochemical studies? J. Histochem. Cytochem. *31*: 244–247 (1983).
27 Huet, B.; Pourriat, J.L.; Martin, J.; Cupa, M.: An automaton computer program for a microcomputerized real-time (thesaurus based) abstract medical record. Comput. Progr. Biomed. *15*: 117–123 (1982).
28 Itoshima, T.; Kawaguchi, K.; Morichika, S.; Ito, T.; Kiyotoshi, S.; Ogawa, H.; Yuasa, S.; Hattori, S.; Kitadai, M.; Ukida, M.; Nagashima, H.: Differential diagnosis of liver parenchymal diseases by likelihood method using 12 laboratory data and age. Gastroenterol. jap. *17*: 453–462 (1982).
29 Itoshima, T.; Kawaguchi, K.; Morichika, S.; Ito, T.; Kiyotoshi, S.; Ogawa, H.; Yuasa, S.; Hattori, S.; Kitadai, M.; Mizutani, S.; Ukida, M.; Nagashima, H.: Ranking of liver tests for differential diagnosis of liver parenchymal diseases. Gastroenterol. jap. *18*: 109–113 (1983).
30 Jagoe, R.; Sowter, C.; Dandy, S.; Slavin, G.: Morphometric study of liver cell nuclei in hepatomas using an interactive computer technique: (i) nuclear size and shape. J. clin. Path. *35*: 1057–1062 (1982).
31 Johannes, R.S.; Cangemi, J.R.; Chesley, J.; Hutcheon, D.F.: A microcomputer system for endoscopic data (Abstract). Gastrointest. Endosc. *29*: 183 (1983).
32 Jost, R.G.; Rodewald, S.S.; Hill, R.L.; Evens, R.G.: A computer system to monitor radiology department activity: a management tool to improve patient care. Radiology *145*: 347–350 (1982).

33 Korman, L.Y.; Johannes, R.S.: Design specifications for a computerized endoscopy database (Abstract). Gastrointest. Endosc. *29*: 193 (1983).
34 Laurent, J.X.: Perendoscopic measurement of gastric pH and use of micro-computer. Acta endosc. *12*: 459–462 (1982).
35 Lindberg, G.; Björkman, A.; Helmers, C.: A description of diagnostic strategies in jaundice. Scand. J. Gastroent. *18*: 257–265 (1983).
36 Llaurado, J.G.: Advances in computer technology: software, hardware and overall perspectives. Int. J. bio-med. Comput. *13*: 361–367 (1982).
37 Lustman, F.: SUMER: A database concept for clinical research and patient data-management. Comput. Prog. Biomed. *15*: 125–132 (1982).
38 MacDonald, R.A.; Pechet, G.S.; Lovenbury, P.: Surgical pathology reports with a portable microcomputer. Archs Pathol. Lab. Med. *106*: 666–669 (1982).
39 Macrae, F.A.; Williams, C.B.: A prospective colonoscopic follow-up study of 500 adenoma patients with multivariate analysis to predict risk of subsequent colorectal tumours (Abstract). Gastroenterology *82*: 1122 (1982).
40 McCloy, R.F.; Vickery, J.C.; Baron, J.H.: Long-term recording and computer analysis of simultaneous gastric and duodenal pH under normal conditions in man. Clin. Phys. Physiol. Meas. *1*: 151–162 (1980).
41 McNeil, B.J.; Pauker, S.G.; Sox, H.C., Jr.; Tversky, A.: On the elicitation of preferences for alternative therapies. New Engl. J. Med. *306*: 1259–1262 (1982).
42 Miller, R.A.; Pople, H.E., Jr.; Myers, J.D.: INTERNIST–1, an experimental computer-based diagnostic consultant for general internal medicine. New Engl. J. Med. *307*: 468–476 (1982).
43 Orlowski, J.; Dodds, W.J.; Linehan, J.H.; Dent, J.; Hogan, W.J.; Arndorfer, R.C.: Requirements for accurate manometric recording of pharyngeal and esophageal peristaltic pressure waves. Investve Radiol. *17*: 567–572 (1982).
44 Pauker, S.G.; Kassirer, J.P.: The threshold approach to clinical decision making. New Engl. J. Med. *302*: 1109–1117 (1980).
45 Pauker, S.G.; Kassirer, J.P.: Clinical decision analysis by personal computer. Archs intern. Med. *141*: 1831–1837 (1981).
46 Ravich, W.J.; Johannes, R.S.; Schneider, W.; Massey, J.T.; Johns, R.J.; Hendrix, T.R.: Portable continuous pH monitoring with computerized data analysis (Abstract). Gastroenterology *84*: 1281 (1983).
47 Reggia, J.A.: Computer-assisted medical decision making: a critical review. Ann. biomed. Eng. *9*: 605–619 (1981).
48 Robboy, S.J.; Altshuler, B.S.; Chen, H.Y.: Retrieval in a computer-assisted pathology encoding and reporting system (CAPER). Am. J. clin. Path. *75*: 654–661 (1981).
49 Rosati, R.A.; McNeer, J.F.; Starmer, C.F.; Mittler, B.S.; Morris, J.J., Jr.; Wallace, A.G.: A new information system for medical practice. Archs intern. Med. *135*: 1017–1024 (1975).
50 Richter, J.M.; Silverstein, M.D.; Schapiro, R.H.: Evaluation of strategies for the diagnosis of suspected obstructive jaundice using clinical decision analysis (Abstract). Gastroenterology *82*: 1161 (1982).
51 Rozen, P.: Computer assitance in gastroenterology: a review. J. clin. Gastroent. *4*: 403–413 (1982).
52 Ryback, R.S.; Eckardt, M.J.; Rawlings, R.R.; Rosenthal, L.S.: Quadratic discriminant

analyis as an aid to interpretive reporting of clinical laboratory tests. J. Am. med. Ass. *248*: 2342–2345 (1982).
53 Saxton, W.O.; Koch, T.L.: Interactive image processing with an offline minicomputer: organization, performance and applications. J. Microsc. *127*: 69–83 (1982).
54 Schichiri, M.; Kawamori, R.; Yamasaki, Y.; Hakui, N.; Abe, H.: Wearable artificial endocrine pancreas with needle-type glucose sensor. Lancet *ii*: 1129–1131 (1982).
55 Summers, R.W.; Cramer, J.; Flatt, A.J.: Computerized analysis of spike burst activity in the small intestine. IEEE Trans. biomed. Engng. *29*: 309–314 (1982).
56 Torchia, M.G.; Cote, D.D.; Danzinger, R.G.: Computer assisted management of total parenteral nutrition (Abstract). Gastroenterology *84*: 1336 (1983).
57 Treat, M.R.; Forde, K.A.: A micro-computer based system for endoscopic data management (Abstract). Gastrointest. Endosc. *29*: 189 (1983).
58 Trell, E.; Dahlberg, N.; Larsson, C.; Krantz, J.-O.; Lazer, A.; Petersson, B.-G.: Interactive computer program for self-distributed medical questionnaire in a population health screening. Comput. Progr. Biomed. *14*: 257–266 (1982).
59 Trell, E.; Dahlberg, N.; Krantz, J.-O.; Larsson, C.; Lazer, A.; Petersson, B.-G.; Åxholt, P.: Experiences with an interactive computer program for recording biometrical health screening data. Comput. Progr. Biomed. *14*: 293–296 (1982).
60 Troxell, R.B.; Kohn, S.R.; Gray, J.W.; Welch, R.W.; Harloe, E.D.; Goyal, R.K.: A computer-assisted technique for 24-hour esophageal monitoring. Dig. Dis. Sci. *27*: 1057–1062 (1982).
61 Vayda, E.; Mindell, W.R.; Mueller, C.B.; Yaffe, B.: Measuring surgical decision-making with hypothetical cases. Can. med. Ass. J. *127*: 287–290 (1982).
62 Weyl, S.; Fries, J.; Wiederhold, G.; Germano, F.: A modular self-describing clinical databank system. Comput. Biomed. Res. *8*: 279–293 (1975).
63 Young, D.W.: A survey of decision-aids for clinicians. Br. med. J. *285*: 1332–1336 (1982).
64 Zajicek, G.; Meinzer, H.P.; Komitowski, D.: Automated image processing of the colon crypt epithelium. Comput. Biomed. Res. *15*: 155–163 (1982).
65 Zeng-lie, L.; Fu-le, H.: Computer-aided diagnosis of gastric cancer. Chin. med. J. *95*: 293–296 (1982).
66 Ziporyn, T.: Computer-assisted medical decision-making: interest growing. J. Am. med. Ass. *248*: 913–918 (1982).

Dr. P. Rozen, Gastroenterology Departement, Ichilov Hospital, 6 Weizman Street, Tel Aviv 64239 (Israel)

Front. gastrointest. Res., vol. 7, pp. 14–26 (Karger, Basel 1984)

An Introduction to Computers

E. Levy[a], *P. Rozen*[b1]

[a]Eddy Levy Scientific and Commercial Programming Company, [b]Municipal-Governmental Medical Center and Sackler Medical School, Tel Aviv, Israel

Introduction

The evolution of the computer is the result of mankind's attempt to solve day-to-day problems speedily and to accomplish tasks beyond our normal capability. It was developed, through the centuries, from mechanical devices which enabled simple computation to the electronic machines of the present era. The computer's rapid development began during World War II., when the need to calculate ballistic data brought about the development of an electronic data processor – or as we today know it, the first computer.

It has developed rapidly from an electromechanical 'counter', through vacuum tube devices into, lately, a device constructed of microscopic-sized printed circuits. These electronics facilitate its high-speed capabilities – including the storage and processing of large quantities of data, the up-date and cancellation of its data, and data transmission over continents, via telephone and satellite communications systems. The computer can perform calculations, comparisons and simulations, as well as serving as a timer for industrial and scientific activities – all carried out easily, speedily, and with high reliability.

Recently, a further major contributing factor to the use of the modern computer has been its marked and continuous decline in cost. This brings the computer within reach of day-to-day applications. This chapter is intended as an introduction, therefore, for non-computer users, explaining and defining simply some of the relevant terminology used in this volume. Further details may be found in pertinent references [1, 2, 4].

[1] The authors are grateful to *T. Cohen* for her assistance in researching this chapter.

What is a Computer?

A computer is an electronic device capable of storing large amounts of information, performing varied arithmetic and logic functions, as well as the efficient handling and editing of data. It receives the data from a source, stores it in its memory system, processes the data, and finally produces the desired output. It is a machine operating at high electronic speeds and functions only according to instructions contained in programs which enable the computer to read, memorize, write, and thus perform many other functions, commercial, industrial and scientific. It is absolutely accurate and objective in taking a position.

Types of Computers

Computers are classified into two main types: The *analog computer* serves for control, production and simulation functions. Input is received in a form of electrical signals which represent measurements of physical phenomena. The input is processed immediately, in *real time*, and the output, which may simulate the phenomena, is received on screens as curves or electrical signals. Until recently, analog computers did not usually store data in large quantities, or have the logic facilities of programmed digital machines. The analog computer has defined uses in clinical medicine, such as data acquisition in many imaging processes. Its other main uses are in laboratories and production processes.

The *digital computer* is used for electronic data processing, or calculating via numbers representing values of variables and quantities. Here the input is quantities, defined digitally, at any desired level of accuracy. It can store data and perform calculations in response to instructions given in the form of a *program*. It is the most commonly used computer, as it answers commercial, scientific and medical needs.

Computer Generations

The development of the computer started with the invention in China of the abacus as a calculating aid, some 5,000 years ago. It enabled simple counting and arithmetic calculations. The development of mechanical calculators and the electromechanical calculation machines was a vital step towards automatic calculation.

In 1890 computer development took a major step forward thanks to the invention of the punch card by Dr. *Herman Hollerith*, a clerk in the American Registration of Inhabitants Office. A tabulator was used to read the data stored on these cards. In 1945, Dr. *Mauchly* of Pennsylvania University designed the ENIAC computer, an electronic device several times faster than any previously known machine. Following this, computer technology was advanced enormously. From the point of view of technological development, generations of computers may be classified as follows:

The First Generation – 1952–1957. This was characterized by the use of vacuum tubes which improved computer speed, and by the development of magnetic memory and storage units.

The Second Generation – 1958–1963. Here solid-state transistors were used to amplify the computer efficiency while reducing its size. Magnetic tapes were also introduced, as cheap and fast external data-storage devices. Computers were also employed in real-time and time-sharing methods, while data analysis was performed by batch processing (see below).

Units designed for a certain computer did not fit another, even if both were from the same manufacturer. Users were in need of a family of compatible computers, where units and programs could be transferred from one computer to another. This brought about the development of the *modular* approach to computer technology which enabled users to enlarge an existing system instead of replacing it with a new system.

The Third Generation – 1964–1969. This was characterized by development of computers where the memory and the arithmetic/logic unit contained *integrated circuits*, which reduced the time and volume of calculations. *Terminals* were introduced and *virtual storage* capability allowed for the execution of programs requiring more memory than actually existed, by storing parts of the data on an external disk and switching between the internal memory and the disk, as necessary. The development of an *operating system*, which controls the computer operation and resources (including the virtual storage) enabled the computer to serve many programs at the same time, *multi-programming*, and perform several functions concurrently, *multi-processing*.

The Fourth Generation – 1970 Onwards. Current computer design employs microscopic-sized integrated circuits etched on silicon chips, which reduces computer size and electricity consumption. Enlargment of the memory capacity is also achieved, as well as advanced mass storage devices. The on-line, immediate processing method has also been developed (see below).

The Computer System

A computer system is comprised of an assembly of equipment units which are called the *hardware.* The units are selected in accordance with the data processing requirements needed, each unit executing a specific function. The hardware responds to a set of written instructions (*programs*) which is called the *software* and operates the equipment.

Thus, the computer system is comprised of software and hardware. A computer system is some arrangement, *configuration*, of machines which are designed and programmed to operate together (fig. 1). When referring to a computer system one should visualize the conversion of data into electronic signals, which pass back and forth between the equipment units of the system via cables, telephone lines or even satellite communication.

Computer Binary Logic. The computer equipment functions through electrical signals, employing the binary code, through use of Boolean algebra. Input and output of the computer utilize the decimal numbers and alphabetical characters (*alphanumeric*) while the internal computer functions are performed with the *binary code.*

A *Boolean argument* may be either true or false. This can be interpreted by an electric device having one of two states, such as in the case of a lamp. An illuminated lamp represents '1' (true) and an extinguished lamp represents '0' (false). Similarly, the computer uses two signs only, and the binary digit (*bit*) is a basic component of any digital computer system. All information is represented by the existence of the binary digit in one of the two possible states. The computer processes digital information by handling groups of bits. 8 bits are needed to encompass and manipulate all the possible characters used, and this is called a *byte.* The sequence of 8 positive or negative signals in the byte (8 bits) is the way any number, symbol, or alphabetic sign is represented in the computer by means of the binary code.

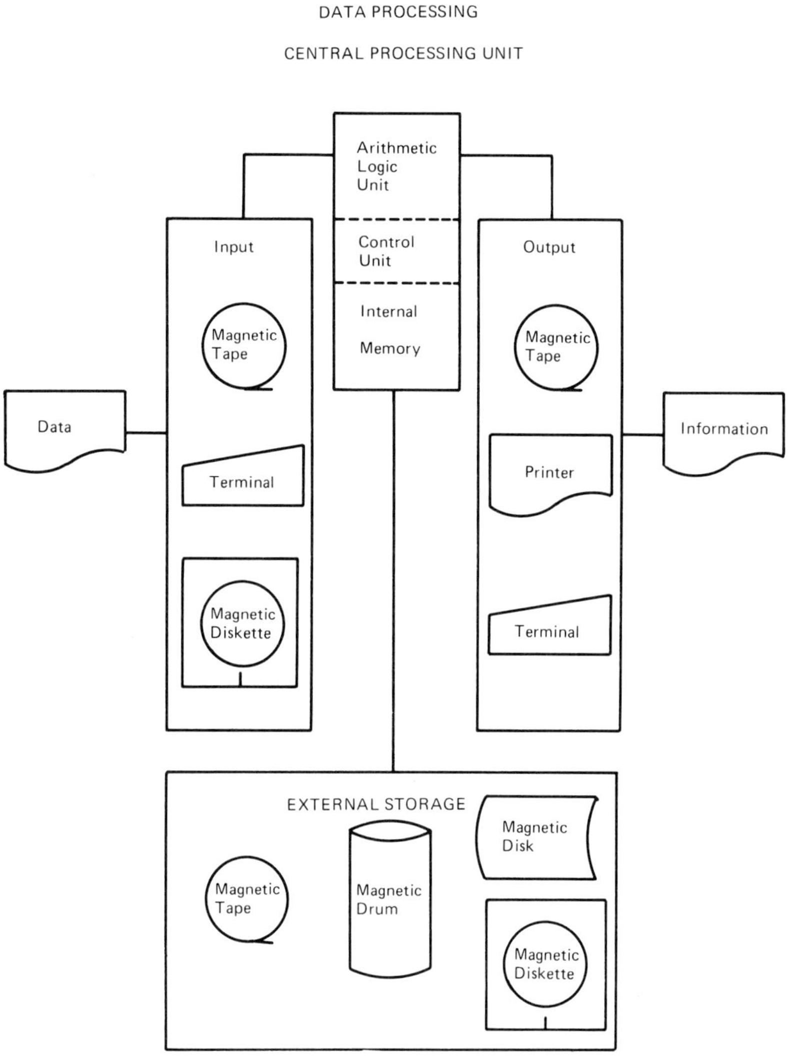

Fig. 1. Schematic arrangement, configuration, of machines (hardware) programmed to operate together.

Thus, when the computer receives the data in the decimal mode, it translates the data into the internal (binary) representation used by the computer through an *encoder*. At termination of the processing, binary numbers are again translated back into decimal numbers by the *decoder*.

Data Processing

Data processing includes receiving data as input, storing the data in one of the memory systems, processing the data, and producing results.

(1) *Input* – data enters the computer directly through a terminal, or from a diskette, magnetic tape, etc. The methods of data processing include: (a) *Batch processing*. Here all instructions and data are gathered and entered as one unit, and then processed continuously by the computer. (b) *On-line processing*. Here data processing is performed in steps. The results of each step is immediately displayed enabling the next step to be performed by addition of data or program parts, and so on. The input and output are connected to the central processing unit.

(2) *Storage* of data is by either of two methods: (a) *Internal memory*. This is sited in the computer's *central processing unit* (CPU) and therefore has a high access speed. (b) *External memory* which may be a magnetic disk, floppy disks, tape or drum. These have low access speed but are capable of storing large amounts of data and because of their less sophisticated construction also cost much less than the internal memory.

(3) *Central processing* – data is transferred to the CPU which is comprised of three parts: (a) *Control unit* – this controls the input units, instructs the arithmetic/logic unit what function to perform, and controls the output units. (b) *Arithmetic/logic unit* – this performs the calculation functions on the data. (c) *Internal memory* – this stores the data to be processed as well as the application program. Time of access to this memory is very short and the data passes at a very high velocity, measurable in nanoseconds. Data is rapidly passed to and from the internal memory and storage units as needed.

There are several types of computer memory, one of which is called *random access memory* (RAM) meaning that it is divided into many compartments each with its own *address* for more rapid direct reference, retrieval and updating of data.

The size of the memory is usually measured in *bytes*. (In most systems a byte can store one character or symbol, and more when used for numeric values only). Because there are thousands or millions of bytes the terms KB (*kilobyte*) and MB (*megabyte*), for a thousand and a million bytes, respectively, are commonly used. They reflect the capability, or power, of the computer system to handling data.

(4) *Output* is produced by a unit such as a printer, terminal, etc.

Software

The term software refers to the entire *assembly of programs* in the computer system. The software designed for a computer system has to match the specific hardware and is divided into two systems: *basic software* and *application program systems*.

Basic Software System

(1) Operating System. This controls the computer work order and the efficient allocation of the computer resources. The type of operating system varies according to the number of users the system can serve simultaneously. *Single programming* is an operating system serving a single program only at a specific time, whilst the *multiprogramming* system serves many programs simultaneously. In this case, the system has to handle allocation of the system resources among the programs it serves simultaneously, especially allocation of the CPU between the programs. This can be achieved by one of two methods: *real time* – where a program may use the CPU only after the previous program terminates its work in the CPU – or *time sharing*. In this latter method the use of the CPU is instantaneously transferred from one program to the other. The operating system arranges a queue for each required resource according to the program input, level of priority, etc. It also controls the programs being simultaneously executed, in order to maintain coordination between them.

(2) Compilers. These are special translating programs which translate programs written in high level languages into machine language. Each computer has a machine language of its own, which is an elementary series of instructions to perform functions by the computer.

(3) Utility Programs. This is a collection, or *library*, of general programs which aids the system user in the management of data files, e.g. sorting, and withdrawal of data, etc.

Application Program Systems

These are programs (generally written in a high level language) executing the instructions and applications for which the computer is intended. This execution is performed through the use of the basic software system and is under its control.

Programming Languages

A computer language instructs the computer how to process data it receives and a program is written by a *programmer* in one or more of these languages. Three types of computer languages are used:

Machine Language. Each computer has its own specific machine language, which is its basic language and is written in binary code. This is an elementary series of instructions to perform functions by the computer.

Symbolic Language. This was developed from the machine language. It uses abbreviated terms written in English letters and thus is more convenient for the user. Each computer has a specific symbolic language of its own. The computer uses an *assembler program* to translate programs and instructions written in symbolic language, to machine language.

High Level Languages. These are general languages compatible with many computers and their use is more recommended than symbolic language. They are very similar to the English language and ease the writing of computer programs. FORTRAN was one of the first high level languages. It is based on algebra and a number of grammar rules, and is intended mainly for scientific applications. Later, languages such as PL/1, BASIC, COBOL and others, were developed for commercial applications.

The development of the high level languages raised the need for translating them to the specific machine language of the computer. This is performed through special translating programs – *compilers*. The *compilation process* consists of translating each high level language instruction into machine language.

Selecting a Computer

The selection of a computer is complex, and first requires an approximate assessment of the computer application needs, preferably by a *systems analyst.* In addition, the consultant must make a comprehensive evaluation of the proposed processing systems and the alternatives, taking into account service reliability, costs and future needs.

Computer applications may be divided into three groups; namely technical, administrative, and scientific applications. When selecting a computer, other factors must be examined in addition to financial considerations. These include the *type of computer*, the *appropriate processing methods* and the *computer operation methods*.

Type of Computer

Computers may be classified by their size into three main groups, namely *mainframe, minicomputer* or *microcomputer*. Frequently, a clear distinction between them cannot be made. The factors that determine the computer capacity are the size of the internal memory and the computer operation speed. Generally, computer design is modular, meaning that the internal memory may be expanded by sections of fixed size, and the basic computer speed can be improved.

(1) Mainframe. This has a large internal memory, usually starting from 1 MB, which may be enlarged as necessary. The mainframe is equipped with a wide variety of peripheral equipment, such as magnetic disks to store a large quantity of data, and other input/output units. Its software system includes a highly sophisticated operating system, backed by a data communication software system, designed for operating a computer network and network activity control. Centralized and large volume processing, requiring many resources, are generally performed by the mainframe.

(2) Minicomputer. A relatively small computer system. Industry, commerce, medical services, etc., have increased their service production impressively by introducing small computer systems. Nowadays, organizations which previously processed data manually, or through a large computer, may purchase minicomputers to perform their applications independently, cheaper, and in a more efficient manner. The minicomputer system is comprised of hardware, software, machine maintenance and support. It is designed in a variety of architectures, and may be enlarged by adding equipment or memories – as required by the user. The user may select one of the following options to cover his requirements: (1) A minicomputer to serve as an independent unit (which is more economical than using a mainframe for small processing purposes). (2) A minicomputer as a component in a computer network (which enables the user to use it independently for his applications while retaining the option of benefitting from the network

resources for his needs). (3) Several minicomputers, each with its own applications at various locations, but acting as one system by connection through a communication network. (Such a system is characterized by high flexibility, efficiency and independence).

(3) Microcomputer. This is a physically small computer which uses one or more *microprocessors*. The extraordinary versatility and productivity of the microcomputer offers a significant new dimension for the role of the computer. The evolving field of inexpensive portable computers has produced a variety of systems (also known as 'personal computers') with speed and memory size similar to some mainframes. Most microcomputers have business applications including accounting and word processing, as well as personal finance and home entertainment applications. The user can begin with a minimum configuration consisting of the microprocessor, keyboard/display, and printer. Later the configuration may be expanded as the task requires, one module at a time.

This expansion capability allows the microcomputer to emerge into large businesses by performing large applications available with commercial software packages. Until recently, their work output was not as great as that provided by the mainframes, since input/output peripherals were not available with microcomputers. However, based on computing speed and cost of computing power, microcomputers are nowadays matching or surpassing the mainframes. Most run a single pogram at a time (no multiprogramming as in mainframes or minicomputers) but provide an individual user with powerful tools.

Processing Methods

The needs of the user are the leading consideration when deciding between *time-sharing* (on-line) and *batch-processing* methods. Some systems necessitate use of a time-sharing method. These systems must have immediate access to the stored data and have a short, immediate, response time.

On the other hand, some systems permit a selection between the two processing methods. When selecting the processing method, one should consider the following factors: (1) The number of simultaneous users; (2) the response time, and (3) the computer applications flexibility.

Hence, where the system is required to be capable of being operated simultaneously by a number of users, to have a short response time, and to provide each user with his individual applications, the time-sharing method is preferred. However, when fast response time is not essential, and processing may be performed in batches, there is no need to invest unnecessary financial resources in computer and communication facilities; the batch-processing method should then be utilized.

Computer Operation Methods

Two systems of operation designs should be considered, *centralized data processing and distributed data processing* (DDP). The choice will depend on the resources and functions required.

Centralized data processing has one, or more, mainframes and all input/output units are connected directly to the central computer, which is an absolutely independent unit. It may be of any type, and it performs the entire processing required, without distribution of its resources.

The *DDP* system is based on a group of local computers which have the possibility of being interconnected through communication lines. The group is generally divided into two types of computers, mainframe or remote computing systems. In the former the mainframes perform the main processing and control the data storage and the network activities. In the remote computer systems, there are local computers connected to the network mainframes, and perform part of the processing. Each computer in the network, central or remote, may be employed as a local computer. The network resources, located at various locations, can serve each computer connected in the network.

This resource sharing has a highly considerable economic advantage, since remote equipment, such as files, programs and program data, may be shared as if they were local resources. A distributed system is less sensitive to failures, since a failure in one particular unit does not influence any other unit in the network. Each may also operate independently of other units in the network.

Computers in Medicine

Computers in medicine were introduced as an answer to *administrative needs*. In the first stage, the computer handled salaries, manpower, financial and medicine inventory subjects, as well as technical follow-up of the patients, insurance company payments and so on. Hospitals that focussed on computer-aided administration achieved impressive performances in management and the administrative service was highly improved; manpower costs were thus reduced [5].

Physicians also – more recently – have studied the application of computers for *diagosis* and *medical treatment*. The computers' capability of storing and processing enormous quantities of data implies it can assist physicians in the diagnosis of a certain disease through employment of an extraordinary large data base [6] [see also *de Dombal*, this volume].

Medical computerization began in hospitals by employing mainframes. These computers were mainly designed for large-scale data-batch processing, while interactive communication was provided only through secondary software packages. However, hospital computerization is characterized by the large number of peripherals needed for accesses to the data base. Employing a mainframe system for these systems does not enable as fast and continuous a response as desired, while the cost is very high. The distributed organization of a hospital, and the problems concerned with mainframe systems, led to the development of *DDP systems* for hospitals. These systems are capable of storing and processing data at several locations, not only in one center.

This system is a *computer network*, generally small computers which are interconnected and tied to a mainframe. Each computer in the network performs a defined and separate function, as desired by the individual department where it is installed. This distributed setup has some significant advantages: (1) It provides a large number of individual accesses to the hospital data reservoirs. By installing a computer network, the response times are shortened, especially because of the reservoir access branching. (2) Each unit in the network is self-contained. Any failure in one of the network computers does not disturb the operation of the other computers in the same network. (3) Each department is autonomous in determining its system development and applications in compliance with its needs. The user has direct and convenient access to the computer. Such a setup advances the software development and makes compliance with the department requirements most efficient [3]. When developing a medical system for a specific department, it can be considered as an independent body, and be developed together with the medical specialists in the field. The system can comply with the needs of the department, independent of the mainframe. (4) By connecting the network to a mainframe, all the administrative and heavy workload processings can be transferred to the mainframe. The mainframe can also store the patient administrative and medical files, etc. This can result in obtaining a standard data base. Each computer in the network can still be capable of operating as an independent unit while using the central data storage for its needs.

Gastroenterology

The research and scientific development of a gastroenterology department requires independent computer resources, providing it with immediate results and responses (in real-time) [7].

Distributed processing in the best method for these requirements, thus guaranteeing the independence of the department, with the ability to communicate with a central computer and transfer data.

A minicomputer with at least a 128–256 KB memory, a 10–64 MB disk (the larger costing less per unit), floppy-disk (diskette) reader; printer (for medical and statistical reports) and several terminals, is a suitable equipment configuation. This type of system, which now serves mainly for data management and research, will be a major tool in the future to assist physicians in patient diagnosis and treatment.

Conclusions

The recent improvements in computer technology, especially the development of small, modular and relatively inexpensive hardware, make it useful for day-to-day applications in medicine. In gastroenterology the computer can aid in data management, research and eventually diagnosis and treatment.

References

1 Chandor, A.; Graham, J.; Williamson, R.: The Penguin dictionary of computers; 2nd ed. (Penguin, Harmondsworth 1981).
2 Davis, G.B.: Management information systems. Conceptual foundation, structure and development (McGraw Hill, New York 1974).
3 Fox, J.: Development of hospital computing. J.R. Soc. Med. *72*: 425–431 (1979).
4 McFayden, J.H.: Systems network architecture. IBM Syst. J. *15*: 4–23 (1976).
5 Norwood, D.D.; Hawkins, R.E.; Gall, J.E., Jr.: Information systems benefits hospital, improves patient care. Hospitals *50*: 79–83 (1976).
6 Rozen, P.: Computer assistance for gastroenterology. A review. Clin. Gastroenterol. *4*: 403–414 (1982).
7 Rozen, P.; Levy, E.; Gilat, T.: Computer assistance for gastrointestinal endoscopy units (Editorial). Gastrointest. Endosc. *28*: 111–112 (1982).

P. Rozen, MD, Gastroenterology Department, Ichilov Hospital, 6 Weizman Street, Tel Aviv 64239 (Israel)

Front. gastrointest. Res., vol. 7, pp. 27–45 (Karger, Basel 1984)

An Overview of Hospital Information Systems: Their Relevance to Gastroenterology

Jeffrey L. Lichtenstein

Yale University Schools of Medicine and Organization and Management, New Haven, Conn., USA

Introduction

'Medical information systems will be the major capital investments of [US] hospitals in the decade of the eighties.' – *Howard Berman*, Vice President of the American Hospital Association, addressing the Eleventh AHA Conference on Hospital Information Systems (1981).

The computer industry in the USA has been growing at an astronomical rate. While computerization in business and industry expanded in earnest in the 1960s and has been moving rapidly ever since, medical applications and installations have been slower to catch on. Recently, however, the health care market in the USA has become too big to ignore. In the past few years computerization in health care, particularly in hospitals, has entered an exponential growth phase.

Whereas hospital expenditures increased in the USA 17% from 1980 to 1981, the portion of the bill for data processing jumped 25% from $1.5 to $1.9 billion [10]. Many hospitals are upgrading their data processing departments with new titles and enhanced status. Departments of Information Systems have replaced Departments of Data Processing. Instead of reporting to the hospital's chief financial officer, many of these department heads now report to the chief executive officer himself. Many are now included in the elite cabinet of top management.

This change reflects a growing enthusiasm for using the computer to organize and integrate the flow of clinical as well as financial information in hospitals. Whereas applications had been limited to accounting and billing for many years, computer systems recently have been developed and aggressively marketed to process clinical information and integrate it with financial and accounting systems.

These new systems go under a confusing array of names and acronyms, both generic and proprietary. The term 'hospital information system' (HIS) will be used here to denote such systems. A HIS can be defined as a computer system that allows different hospital departments to communicate with each other and to update and access a shared data base (or set of data bases) of clinical and administrative information.

There are now many companies, small and large, marketing such systems in the USA. Many are new and compensate for their limited track record with low prices and unbounded promises. Some are established hardware manufacturers, such as IBM and Burroughs, who have developed systems specifically for their machines. Most companies, however, are software developers and consultants.

Development of the first true HIS began in 1965 at El Camino Hospital in Mountain View, Calif. The hospital started the project in conjunction with Lockhead Corporation. Technicon acquired Lockhead's health care data processing operation in 1971 and installed an operational system at El Camino in 1972.

The system achieved prominence after the National Center for Health Services Research (NCHSR) contracted with the Battelle Corporation to prepare a comprehensive evaluation of the El Camino system [9].

Although a variety of hardware improvements and software efficiencies have been introduced, there have been no stunning innovations beyond the original El Camino system. Cost is now lower, reliability is greater, and some new functions and departments have been added to the system [4]. Although the latest hardware and software configurations are often technically different, operationally the functions of today's systems are remarkably similar to the original El Camino system.

To date, no commerically successful HIS can replace the paper medical record for inpatients. Furthermore, none are specifically designed to aid in diagnosis, to analyze data for research, or to educate clinicians about medical advances. Unlike some of the computer applications discussed in other chapters, the primary goals of HIS are to facilitate communication among hospital departments, to maintain computerized records of selected clinical information (such as the results of a laboratory tests) and to generate bills.

Touring a Computerized Hospital

In order to better understand how a HIS affects the traditional functions of a hospital, it will be useful to follow a hypothetical patient through a computerized hospital. Dr. *Core* sees a patient, Mrs. *Stein*, in his office with severe chest pain. He arranges for immediate hospital admission. Because Mrs. *Stein* has been a patient at the hospital before, the admission clerk can display her demographic and insurance information on the computer terminal screen simply by entering her name. The clerk asks the patient or family if the information is still correct, makes any changes, then tells the computer to admit the patient. Bed assignment is accomplished quickly and easily. Dr. *Core* has requested a coronary care unit (CCU) bed, the current status of beds in the CCU is instantly displayed and the clerk assigns a bed to Mrs. *Stein*.

The computer then alerts the CCU that Mrs. *Stein* is to be admitted with a diagnosis of possible myocardial infarction. With the addition of Mrs. *Stein*, however, there are too few nurses in the CCU to adequately meet the needs of the patients. At her terminal, the nursing supervisor checks the roster of nurses who have CCU qualifications. She can quickly check their assignments and schedules and make the most appropriate choice of an additional nurse to rotate into the CCU.

Dr. *Core* calls in his admission orders to the CCU nurse who enters them into her computer terminal. When Mrs. *Stein* arrives, the orders are activated. The computer notifies the laboratory that immediate, STAT blood work must be drawn in the CCU, notifies the X-ray Department that a portable chest X-ray must be taken, notifies EKG that a STAT cardiogram is to be done, notifies the kitchen to send up a meal, notifies pharmacy about the drugs ordered, etc. The computer eliminates repetitive telephone dialing, busy signals, garbled messages, 'lost' orders, and late orders.

Furthermore, once an order is placed, the computer can remember it and remind the staff about it until it is either completed or cancelled. The CCU can find out the status of an order by simply inquiring at the terminal. For example, the nurse can quickly find out whether blood was received in the laboratory for the tests ordered and whether or not results are ready.

As soon as the laboratory or X-ray completes the tests ordered, the computer prints the results in the CCU. The information is transferred reliably, quickly, and accurately without the frustrations of making a telephone connection or the inaccuracies of transferring numerical data from paper to mouth to ear to paper. The nurse knows the computer does not need to be prompted and will send the results as soon as they are ready, eliminating unnecessary calls to the laboratory.

At the same time the laboratory result is reported to the floor, the computer updates Mrs. *Stein*'s bill with the appropriate charges for those laboratory tests. Multicarbon forms no longer need to be shuffled from department to department. Patients are billed only for services received and lost charges are eliminated. Furthermore, with the introduction of printed bar code labels for hospital supplies (such as urethral catheter sets) that can be read by light pen and entered into the computer, inventory can be more easily maintained and charges can be recorded which would not be feasible to record in a manual system.

Although many doctors prefer to write their orders on paper, Dr. *Core* usually enters his orders directly at the terminal. Before the computer transmits the orders to the appropriate departments, the head nurse checks them at her terminal. This ensures good communication with the floor and assures accuracy. Nurses' notes and patients vital signs are entered into the computer. Record keeping is easier, quicker, and more legible. The computer also helps with the formulation of a nursing care plan.

On a regular basis the CCUs printer produces a laboratory and medication flow sheets for Mrs. *Stein*. After 3 days her cardiac enzymes have remained normal. Dr. *Core* decides to transfer her to a regular department and seeks a consultation from Dr. *Ramhorn*, a gastroenterologist.

The computer notifies the admitting office of the transfer. Although there are several open beds on one medical ward, there are none available for a woman. The admitting clerk discusses the possibilities of room swapping with the head nurse on the medical ward. Both of them refer to the computer's census report for that floor. They plan a complex swap of male and female patients, which frees a room for Mrs. *Stein*. The switchboard, the information desk, and the mail room are notified of the new room assignments and a STAT work order is placed with housekeeping.

When Dr. *Ramhorn* arrives in the hospital, he punches in at the computer terminal in the doctor's coat room. He is presented with a printed list of his currently hospitalized patients sorted by room number. In addition, a message is displayed for him to examine Mrs. *Stein* as a consultant. The switchboard is alerted that Dr. *Ramhorn* is now in the hospital.

Dr. *Ramhorn* orders an oral cholecystogram and barium meal for Mrs. *Stein*. X-ray is notified; the clerk in X-ray reviews the schedule for the following day and assigns Mrs. *Stein* a time. The computer then automatically notifies pharmacy to send iopanic acid (Telepaque) tablets to the floor that evening and notifies the kitchen that Mrs. *Stein* should not receive breakfast.

When the pharmacy receives the order for iopanic acid tablets, the computer automatically searches for drug/drug or drug/patient incompatibilities. Mrs. *Stein* is allergic to iodinated compounds. The computer alerts the pharmacist who calls Dr. *Ramhorn*. He cancels the oral cholecystogram and orders an ultrasound examination. In addition to notifying X-ray of the change, the computer prompts the clerk to be sure that the ultrasound is scheduled to be performed before the previously ordered barium meal.

Needless to say, gallstones are discovered, and Mrs. *Stein* is booked for surgery. Scheduling in the operating room is greatly facilitated by the computer.

Two weeks after admission, Mrs. *Stein* is ready for discharge. The computer prints her discharge medication prescriptions and instructions. Her bill is ready at the business office with all the appropriate allowances for insurance coverage deducted. Her insurance company is, of course, automatically billed. Dr. *Bite*, her surgeon, dictates a discharge summary, a chore made easier with the computer-generated flow charts of data in the record. After discharge, key information about her hospital stay is retained on file by the computer.

HIS Subsystems

The effect of a HIS is intended to be more than the sum of its parts. Whereas automation of one or two functions might be interesting, it would not appreciably change the way people do their jobs. Furthermore, the quality of the work they do might change only marginally. The real benefit of an HIS comes with the *integration* of many functions. The computer is not only a data repository but it is also a dispatcher and monitor of information. Ideally, it automatically notifies those who need to know what they need to know when they need to know it. At the same time, it monitors information for completeness and consistency.

To function effectively as a dispatcher, however, the computer needs a wide scope of operations. If only one or two departments or functions are included, the power of message switching and communications, as well as the completeness of the data base, are seriously diminished. Staff have to remember what is on the system and what is off, what to enter at a terminal and what not to, when to telephone for results and when to wait for a printout.

Hospitals perform a myriad of functions. Table I is a partial list of the hospital functions that have been commercially developed as subsystems

Table I. HIS subsystems

Admissions, discharges, and transfers	Radiology scheduling
Accounting and general ledger	Nursing notes and care plan
Billing	Nurse staffing
Payroll and personnel	Outpatient scheduling
Order entry	Utilization review
Results reporting	Equipment maintenance schedule
Patient data base update and retrievence	Disease and operations index preparation
Dietary master list	Discharge analysis
Emergency room registration/data base linkage	Tumor registry
Laboratory work schedules and specimen pickup schedules	Medical staff privileges and activities reporting
Pharmacy drug profiles and compatability checks	Supplies inventory
Poison control and antidotes	Housekeeping management
Operating room/recovery room management	Laundry management

of available HISs. There are three subsystems, however, that are often regarded as the core of a HIS: admissions, discharges, and transfers (ADT); accounting and finance; and order entry/results reporting (OE/(RR).

One inpatient stay is the fundamental transaction of the hospital. To record the beginning and ending of each hospitalization is the sine qua non of the HIS. The ADT subsystem performs this function. The admitting office opens or reactivates a patient's computer file using the ADT subsystem. All other information captured during the hospitalization is then entered or indexed in that file. The ADT subsystem keeps track of the patients' current location in the hospital which allows reports about the patient to be sent to the proper place. When the patient is discharged, the transaction is complete and the ADT subsystem prompts other subsystems to perform their functions, such as preparing the bill.

Little needs to be said here about accounting and financial subsystems. Most moderate and large institutions computerized their business offices long ago. HIS vendors now recognize the importance of linking existing financial systems to their new products. Linked to an HIS, much of the billing process can be automated, which cuts down on clerical tasks and reduces billing mistakes.

If ADT is the backbone of the HIS, OE/RR are the muscles. Order entry is the ability to enter orders from the nursing station. Results reporting is ability to receive results (e.g. laboratory results) at the nursing station. Although the two appear to go hand and hand, they represent different levels of software sophistication. Whereas 21 of 24 HIS vendors surveyed by the NCHSR in 1981 offered order entry, only 13 had results reporting systems available [13]. In spite of software distinctions, the logic of hospital operations tie the two together hand in hand. Order entry – which is easier to implement – appears to have much less impact on nursing efficiency than the combination. By and large, conventional manual systems are much more efficient at transmitting orders than at reporting results. Since much of the pinpointed savings engineered by HISs come from improved nursing efficiency, combining order entry and results reporting should assume high priority for most institutions contemplating a HIS installation.

These three subsystems – ADT, accounting and finance, and OE/RR – form the core of a HIS. In addition to this core, a large selection of other subsystems are commercially available. Although none are specifically designed for gastroenterologists, gastroenterology wards, or endoscopy services, many would seem applicable or adaptable.

The pathology laboratory is a major subsystem. Many hospitals with no other clinical computer application have a laboratory system. There are many self-contained laboratory systems that provide a range of functions from transforming analog autoanalyzer signals to printed laboratory results, to word processing for pathology reports. When linked to a HIS, however, the power of a laboratory subsystem can dramatically increase. From the clinician's point of view, the most important benefits are reduced turn around time and flow charting of results. Furthermore, the ability to check easily on the status of a test ordered can reduce frustration immeasurably. For example, a gastroenterologist who orders a serum gastrin or anti-mitochondrial antibody, which is ordinarily shipped to a outside laboratory, can easily find out from the computer whether and when the sample was sent and whether the results have arrived. Furthermore, with a laboratory subsystem, preadmission test results are less likely to be lost or delayed in reaching the chart.

A pharmacy subsystem can play a useful role in keeping track of the polypharmacy of most chronically ill patients. By screening for drug interactions and incompatibilities, the computer can remind the clinician, for example, that aminophylline dosages may have to be reduced after the patient begins taking cimetidine, or that a patient with a cefazolin prescription is allergic to penicillin. Legible flow sheets of medications, dosages, and times may prove quite useful in ferreting out the cause of unexplained fever or diarrhea.

An ongoing computerized patient data base that includes relevant information from each hospitalization is available with most commercial HISs. The amount and type of information that can be stored will vary from system to system. Some systems will be more flexible than others in terms of the arrangement of data in the stored files and the way the data can be retrieved. As a minimum, the system should be able to rapidly retrieve an individual patient file and display its contents. This facility could be very useful when confronted with a sick patient in the emergency room or a tall stack of old charts.

A more sophisticated HIS will allow analysis of subsets of the entire patient data base. Descriptive statistics can be generated to characterize the type of patients treated, clinical outcome of care, resources used, etc. In addition, physicians can be compared in their use of the hospital and its resources.

One of the more promising uses of HISs for the gastroenterologist is for scheduling and logging gastrointestinal procedures. Software that has been developed for use in X-ray departments and operating room suites should be easily adaptable for endoscopic units and gastrointestinal laboratories. Scheduling of procedures can be facilitated with an on-line booking system; a daily schedule can be printed out. A computerized log of room utilization and type of procedure can be quite helpful in improving management of the facility and planning future services. An integrated system can also allow for tracking of biopsy reports and X-ray results. Utilization statistics by physician can be enhanced by reports describing the frequency and types of diagnosis made.

Equipment maintenance records can also be part of many HISs. Preventive maintenance schedules can be generated as well as records of repair and time lost. These may be helpful not only in enhancing equipment safety and life, but in planning future purchases.

Although HISs are primarily designed for inpatients, most vendors can integrate outpatient data and provide services for outpatient departments. This is crucial for a gastroenterology laboratory, which, like X-ray, has a free mix of inpatients and outpatients. In a hospital with many outpatient clinics, patients are often faced with a confusing assortment of appointments. Without a computerized scheduling system it becomes almost impossible to coordinate multiple appointments to different clinics and services. This fosters broken appointments, 'no shows', overbooking, and underbooking. The result is unhappy patients, frustrated staff, and reduced quality of care. Streamlining and computerizing the process improve its efficiency and quality.

Systems and Suppliers

Ten years ago, a hospital that wanted to develop a comprehensive information system probably would have decided to hire programmers and develop the system from scratch. In fact, a few hospitals, undaunted by the complexity and cost of the project, did so. Often they collaborated with an outside consultant or hardware manufacturer. The outside firm bore some of the development costs in return for marketing rights to the system. A heavy investment in time and money on both sides was inevitable; results, on the other hand, were unpredictable.

The industry has matured considerably since then. Although some hospitals still elect to custum design their own systems, most do not. Vendors have packaged services and products to appeal to hospitals at all levels of technical sophistication. At one level, experienced software consultants will work with hospital programmers to custom tailor a system unique to the institution. On another level, it is possible to purchase a ready made system to be installed and maintained with no technical input from the hospital. Most HIS vendors have developed a set of basic software with enough flexibility and optional features that it can be readily tailored to fit most institutions. The vendor usually supplies hardware, software, and some technical training for the hospital's data processing staff.

Hardware can range from a large off-site mainframe computer which is shared by a number of institutions to a distributed network of mini- and microcomputers located within each department of the hospital. Most systems, however, are based on an in-house mainframe or minicomputer.

Software can range from a ready made package of programs in a 'turn key' system to a design that virtually starts from scratch. The system and software can be fully maintained and operated by the vendor with a service bureau or facilities management arrangement, or the hospital can own, maintain, and operate the system independently. Most vendors, however, protect their software and will not provide full documentation of their computer programs. The software may allow a limited number of program modifications to be performed by hospital personnel, but major modifications or troubleshooting must be done by the vendor. Such an arrangement forces the hospital to contract with the vendor for maintenance.

Described below are several HIS vendors. They more or less represent the ever growing number of companies in the HIS field. The field is changing rapidly and the reader is urged to make his own survey.

Technicon Medical Information Systems Corporation (Santa Clara, Calif.). Technicon pioneered the commercial concept of hospital information systems and despite heavy competition has remained an industry leader. It appears to be a well-managed aggressive company and has grown exponentially in recent years. In 1980, it was acquired by Revlon and now has over 70 systems installed.

Several years ago, a hospital could only buy a complete HIS package from Technicon. With a choice of all or nothing, many potential customers chose nothing. The Technicon system is now modular. It can be installed in a stepwise fashion. Furthermore, Technicon can now interface its system with many existing hospital computers. If a hospital already has a satisfactory billing and accounting system, for example, Technicon can tailor its system to fit around and communicate with the existing system.

Technicon works with hospital data processing staff to plan carefully the implementation of their system. Hospital employees become involved in the process early and work side by side with a team from Technicon. After installation, Technicon works alongside hospital staff to maintain the system.

The system is based on a mainframe computer, such as an IBM 4300, which can be located on-site or off-site. Most functions are on-line with intelligent terminals. The cost of the system varies but appears to be of the order of $4.00 per patient per day for a moderately large institution.

HBO & Company (Atlanta, Ga.). This company has become a major vendor with about 300 systems installed. Like Technicon, their approach is modular. They will, however, install and maintain their system without technical support from the hospital. In essence, HBO can function in place of an inhouse data processing department. Their system uses on-site minicomputers such as Hewlett Packard HP 3000.

IBM (General Systems Division, Coral Gables, Fla.). For many years, IBM has been the mainstay of the traditional data processing market in hospitals. Most of its installations consist of hardware and standard business software to support payroll, accounting, billing and other administrative functions. Recently, however, IBM has entered the HIS software market and have developed and supported a number of software systems to run on their hardware.

One such software system is the Hospital Patient Management System (HPMS) designed for small and medium-size hospitals. It is a licensed software program available through IBM, for a monthly fee, that runs on the IBM system/34. The hospital is solely responsible for the successful implementation and maintenance of the system.

Other HIS packages are available through IBM, such as the IBM Patient Care System designed for hospitals over 200 beds. A HIS based on the new IBM System/38 is being developed. Because many hospital data processing managers are loyal IBM users, software marketed and supported by IBM will probably capture an increasing share of the HIS market.

IBM has an active users group known as ECHO (Electronic Computing Health Oriented). It meets semiannually to exchange information and publishes monthly a newsletter called *Boondocks*.

Shared Medical Systems Corporation (King of Prussia, Pa.). Shared Medical Systems (SMS) was founded in 1969 to act as a computer service bureau for the health care industry. Using its mainframe computer in King of Prussia, it focussed on off-site data processing for medical records and financial applications. The majority of its business is still in these two areas, but SMS is now aggressively marketing a group of applications that nest together to form a comprehensive HIS.

The SMS system runs on in-hospital minicomputers which must be linked to the large SMS host computer in King of Prussia. They offer hospitals a turn-key system; installation and maintenance are all done by SMS without technical input from the hospital.

SMS has established an international corporation, SMS International, to market systems outside North America.

Discussion

There is no question that HISs (as they are currently marketed in the USA) will bring a substantial change in the ethos of health care institutions. Data processors will become 'Information specialists' and clerks will become 'computer operators'. Terminals and printers will replace telephones and scraps of paper. Nursing stations will resemble airline ticket counters. Everyone will become more dependent on the machine, than on each other, for their information.

Like industry, hospitals must keep up with the computer revolution. In our society, high technology stands for superior health care and the computer is the icon of high technology. A computer terminal in the admitting office or at the nursing station serves as the centerpiece of white formica and tinted glass altars to technology. It conveys reassurance to patients and providers alike. It says subliminally but forcefully: this is a modern hospital that has the latest technology and therefore the best care.

The commercial success of HISs may be as much a function of their enormous symbolic value as their tangible benefits. In spite of the impressive a priori arguments for tangible benefits from HISs, these benefits have been difficult to document. There are three major types of benefits that a computerized system might achieve: efficiency, management control, and quality of care.

Efficiency. Until recently, HIS vendors promised cost benefit above all else for their systems. Automation of clerical functions would reduce the need for clerks; less recordkeeping for nurses would improve productivity; in short, fewer personnel would be needed for the same level of activity.

Estimates of savings in personnel, however, have been vastly overstated [2, 6]. No HIS has been more extensively studied than the El Camino Hospital system. Excluding the cost of the computer system, no significant change in cost per patient could be detected [3]. Although nursing costs per admission declined by 5%, these changes were offset by rises in the costs of ancillary services. Furthermore, the reduction in nursing cost per admission was largely due to a reduced length of stay per patient. Although the HIS may have been a factor in length of stay reduction, it seems likely that other factors – including the Hawthorne effect (i.e. a placebo effect of any positive change in working conditions) – might have been as important if not more important. When the cost of the system is added in, cost benefit becomes negative.

Why should this be so? Doesn't the computer simplify clerical tasks? Aren't complex communications improved? Aren't errors reduced? Isn't scheduling more efficient? All of the above are probably true, but the facts of organizational life and the current design of work introduce substantial friction that drags down theoretical estimates of personnel savings. Reducing the workload of a full-time ward clerk at a nursing station by 10% doesn't translate into actual savings of 200 man hours per year. Instead, the ward clerk now has 5 or 6 more minutes per hour to do her job. Ward clerks are not exempt from Parkinson's law: work expands to fill the time available for its completion.

In order to realize a savings in personnel, the computer must fully replace a person. Saving one tenth of 10 people's jobs does not add up to saving one whole job. Improved productivity must add up to fewer people in order to save money. A marginal reduction in workload for an employee does not necessarily reduce costs or improve his performance.

In light of this, some vendors have toned down their claims for savings in personnel. It is now said that the HIS will not reduce existing personnel; instead it will allow expansion of volume with fewer additional personnel. Although the El Camino study suggested small overall cost increase per patient despite substantial volume increases [3], the point is difficult to document. To an administrator who is already decided on a HIS, however, the rationale of labor savings with growth is attractive, and is unlikely to be conclusively proven wrong.

Another claim is that employee job satisfaction increases with computerization. Improved job satisfaction may result in improved employee recruitment and retention. The problem of employee turnover, particularly in nursing, vexes most hospital administrators in the USA. Although the nurses at El Camino Hospital have had a favorable response to their HIS [4, 9], there are scarce date documenting effects on turnover. On the other hand, for each story of employee enthusiasm with a new computer system, there seems to be another anecdote of employee frustration and revolt [5].

Employee acceptance seems to be a function of the quality and 'user friendliness' of the system, the degree of user participation in the planning process, the institutional commitment to the system, and the quality of training and support for new system users. A successful installation therefore requires a major mobilization of institutional resources. Money alone will not buy a successful system. The necessary planning and discussion at all levels of an institution requires an enormous commitment of time and personnel. Reorganization of management responsibilities may disrupt the organization before compensating benefits are realized.

Capture of lost charges is another off-cited benefit of HISs [6]. In the hubbub of everyday activities, patients are not always charged for all the services they receive. A hospitalization may consist of hundreds of transactions in different departments, each of which should be itemized on the final bill. It's no wonder that in many institutions 5% or more of charges are never captured on the patient bill. Because the computer captures each transaction as it happens (or as the results are reported), patients are billed accurately for all the services they receive.

The effect could be substantial if hospital reimbursement in the USA were straightforward. An extra dollar on the patient's bill, however, usually does not mean an extra dollar in the hospital coffers. Most patients in US hospitals are covered by insurance that pays costs, not charges. Although an itemized bill is generated with charges tallied up, its use is only indirect in working out how much the hospital is to be paid by the insurance company. Periodically hospital and insurance company accountants get together to perform cost studies to determine what the hospital's cost of doing business is and what proportion of the total cost should be borne by that insurance company. Where reimbursement is based on costs rather than charges, revenue is not necessarily lost when charges are lost. It is only when a charge is lost for the minority of patients (or insurance companies) who pay charges instead of costs that revenue is lost.

Management Control. In the business world, the term 'management information systems' is giving way to the term 'decision support system'. This change reflects a new emphasis on the use of computer systems by management to aid in long-range as well as day-to-day decision making. Data is not only compiled and stored, but selected and analyzed. To be a 'decision support system', the information system should do more than type reports, automate bookkeeping, and send messages. It should be able to select data from a variety or sources, analyze it, and produce reports that aid high-level managers and chief executives in making important or dificult decisions.

HISs as they are currently marketed are not 'decision support systems'. Although the computer may be crammed with data on every aspect of hospital operations, few systems can produce more than simple reports with crude statistics. The heart of the problem is not software, but is conceptual.

Whereas businesses carefully define their markets and their products, most hospitals do not. Although cost per patient day or employees per admission are sometimes used as measures of hospital performance, they are too crude even for gross comparisons among hospitals. Internal management and control requires much more sophistication in defining measures of performance.

A day in the hospital or a discharged patient is an inadequate definition of what a hospital produces. It is too heterogeneous and too crude. A day in an intensive care unit attached to a respirator is very different from a day in a psychiatric ward with group therapy. A hospitalization for coronary bypass surgery is very different in kind and cost from a hospitalization for a normal vaginal delivery.

Until recently it was impossible to define these differences in a systematic and useful way. A means now exists to account for these clinical differences. It is a system of patient classification that defines 467 diagnosis-related groups, 'DRGs' [7, 8]. Each patient discharged from the hospital can be assigned to one of the DRGs based on age, discharge diagnosis, and surgical procedures. The information required to classify patients is part of the standard discharge abstract compiled by US hospitals.

A DRG represents a group of patients who are clinically similar in that they can be expected to consume similar types and amounts of hospital resources. For example, there is one DRG for patients with gastrointestinal hemorrhage who do not require surgery and who do not have significant comorbid disease, such as congestive heart failure.

Each DRG can be considered a type of product that the hospital produces. Discharge of a patient in a particular DRG represents the production of one of those products. A hospital can be thought of as producing 467 product types.

Hospitals can calculate an average cost for each DRG. Meaningful cost comparisions can then be made among hospitals. Since the groups are clinically meaningful, physicians and administrators can begin to dissect out the causes for wide variations in costs among hospitals.

More importantly, DRGs can be used as the cornerstone of an internal management information system. Hospital management can begin to understand what it costs to produce its products, and why costs are what they are. The effects of management decisions about new equipment, new procedures, or new personnel can be measured and monitored. A hospital's mix of products, or case mix, can be defined and conscious decisions about future growth and its effect on operations and 'profitability' can be made.

The use of DRGs is in its infancy. Using DRGs as a tool to analyze the wealth of operational data compiled by the HIS, perspicacious administrators and physicians may usher the dawn of a new era of hospital management and control.

Quality of Care. This is an elusive concept to measure. It seems attractive to say that a HIS will improve patient care by improving efficiency in scheduling, accuracy and timeliness of results reporting, cross-checking of allergies and drug interactions, etc. The actual effect on patient care is difficult to assess and almost impossible to quantify.

Part of the reason that improvement is difficult to demonstrate is that existing manual hospital procedures are not grossly inadequate or inaccurate. Many effective cross-checking mechanisms have evolved. Doctor's orders are reviewed by a professional nurse who bears a legal as well as moral responsibility to question an order that appears to be inappropriate or erroneous. Although laboratory results are occasionally misplaced or delayed, serious problems are unusual in US hospitals. Hospital laboratory performancy is vigorously monitored and certified by the College of American Pathologists and the Joint Commission for the Accreditation of Hospitals. Furthermore, few medical staff would tolerate more than occasional delays or errors in the collection of laboratory specimens or the reporting of results. Although a computer system may speed things up a bit, it is doubtful that a substantial improvement in patient care would result.

Customary hospital practice includes a multitiered system for checking drug allergies and incompatibilities. As a matter of routine, both nurse and doctor ask about drug allergies. When an allergy is uncovered, the chart, the nurses, card index and the medication sheet are labeled in bright colors. In addition to physicians, pharmacists are attuned to the possibilities of adverse interactions among drugs. In many hospital pharmacies a drug profile is manually maintained on each patient. The pharmacist will inform the physician if a potentially dangerous combination is noted. Occasional errors may occur, and no system, whether computer-based or not, can prevent them all. Fortunately, the few errors that do occur rarely have serious untoward effects.

The ability of the computer to arrange information in particular formats (e.g. chronological flow charts of laboratory tests) is a useful feature. It especially aids consultants to rapidly review complex cases. It is doubtful, however, that the end result is an improved outcome for the patient. Under the less elegant old system, the doctor may have to work harder for the information, but his professionalism demands that he glean the necessary data.

The problem-oriented medical record developed by *Weed* [12] is to date the most comprehensive attempt to improve quality of care by improving the format of recordkeeping. A cadre of dedicated supporters has vigorously applied *Weed*'s [12] ideas. None the less, the problem-oriented record has yet to convincingly demonstrate improvement in quality of patient care.

Supported by the NCHSR, *Weed* and collegues have developed a computerized information system known as PROMIS for problem-oriented medical information system. An evaluation of PROMIS versus a non-computerized problem-oriented system was conducted at the Medical Center

Hospital of Vermont by an independent team sponsored by NCHSR [11]. They compared an experimental PROMIS ward with a manual problem-oriented ward at the same hospital. They found no difference in clinically relevant problems identified or in clinically relevant tests or procedures ordered. A panel of physicians made a blinded comparison of matched PROMIS and manual charts. They found that the computer-generated PROMIS records were less concise and had a poorer organization of content. Furthermore, a study of user acceptance of the PROMIS system found that despite enthusiasm for the system in principle, users were ambivalent in practice. The study concluded that the computerized PROMIS system 'neither enhanced nor detracted from patient care'.

The patient data base contained in the HIS could play a useful role to screen and monitor potential problems in clinical care. The HIS could indirectly improve quality by making it easier to compare patterns of care among practitioners and to identify questionable practices and outcomes. The data base could be periodically screened for possible problems such as single unit blood transfusions, antibiotic use without prior cultures, or high proportions of appendectomy with normal appendix. Unfortunately, such uses of HIS patient data bases are not widely used or well developed.

A system of quality assurance screening which uses the more limited data of discharge abstracts has been developed by the Commission of Professional Hospital Activities (CPHA, Ann Arbor, Mich.). It is known as the Quality Assurance Monitor, and is available to hospitals that subscribe to their discharge analysis service (PAS). Unfortunately, as of now, CPHA services cannot be directly linked to HIS patient data bases.

The major impediment to using HIS-generated data for quality assurance work is the lack of sophisticated analysis or report generating capabilities as part of most HIS software. By and large HISs are not designed to allow the data base to be managed easily or efficiently. Reports are generally available only in standardized formats. Analysis is usually confined to simple sorting of small subsets of data. Thus, despite the ability of HISs to generate an extensive clinical data base, available systems are not yet capable of exploiting it fully for quality assurance work.

Conclusions

HISs are expensive, difficult and disruptive to install and have modest tangible benefits. But hospitals will continue to buy them because of the enormous appeal and promise of computer technology. Physicians and administrators want to be part of the computer revolution; they are afraid of being left behind. Computers promise dramatic changes and dazzle even the jaded observer.

As currently designed, however, HISs do not live up to their promise; they merely do by machine what men can do by hand. They are marginally faster, neater and more accurate, but they are not revolutionary.

To date, HIS development has imitated and refined the early success of the El Camino Hospital system. The systems use the computer to imitate what clerks, nurses and technicians do with pens, forms, and telephones. This achievement has been important but in order to be revolutionary, the power of the computer should be used to create new ways to operate hospitals. The work of the hospital must be redefined. The functions of doctors, nurses, clerks, administrators, and the ever-growing array of technicians and paraclinicians should be rethought and redesigned to make use of the computer's potential. More attention should be paid in hospitals to what businesses are learning about their computer information systems [1]. Having the computer do what man cannot, will revolutionize hospital practice. With care and thought, the change will be for the better.

Despite their current limitations, however, the deployment of HISs is a necessary first step in the evolution of the hospital of the future. As physicians, administrators, and hospital staff become at ease with the computer, they will demand more from it. They will be prepared for new developments in voice recognition and artificial intelligence. They will be ready for new applications and create a market for them.

Few of the available HISs deal specifically with the field of gastroenterology but touch it peripherally. Some may be adapted to cope with this subspecialty, while in the future subsystems may be prepared specifically.

By working with the technology as it now exists, hospitals will become sophisticated enough to look for new ways to exploit their information systems. Working with programmers and vendors, hospitals will muster the creativity to redesign the future.

References

1 Allen, B.: An unmanaged computer system can stop you dead. Harvard Bus. Rev. *60*: 76–87 (1982).

2 Bush, I.E.: Trouble with medical computers. Perspect. Biol. Med. *22*: 600–620 (1979).

3 Coffey, R.M.: How a medical information system affects hospital costs: the El Camino hospital experience, HCNSR Research Summary Series. DHEW Publication No. (PHS) 80–3265 (National Center for Health Services Research, Hyattsville 1980).
4 Cook, M.; Fleming, J.J.; Buchanan, N.S.: El Camino Hospital: ten years later. Comput. Hosp. *2*: 22–25 (1981).
5 Dowling, A.F., Jr.: Do hospital staff interfere with computer system implementation? Hlth Care Mgmnt Rev. *5*: 23–32 (1980).
6 Drazen, E.; Metzger, J.: Methods for evaluating costs of automated hospital information systems, NCHSR Research Summary Series. DHHS Publication No. (PHS) 81–3283 (National Center for Health Services Research, Hyattsville 1980).
7 Fetter, R.B.: The new ICD-9CM diagnosis-related groups classification scheme, final report. Hlth Care Financing Administration Grant Nos. 95P97499/1–01 and 95P97491/1–02 (Yale Health Systems Management Group, New Haven 1982).
8 Fetter, R.B.; Shin, Y.; Freeman, J.L.; Averill, R.F.; Thompson, J.D.: Case-mix definition by diagnosis-related groups. Med. Care *18*: suppl., pp. 1–53 (1980).
9 Gall, J.E., Jr.; Norwood, D.D.: Demonstration and evaluation of a total information system, NCHSR Research Summary Series. DHEW Publication No. (HRA) 77–3188 (National Center for Health Services Research, Hyattsville 1977).
10 Oveson, D.A.: Data processing in hospitals, a $1,885,000,000 market. Comput. Hlthcare *3*: 58–59 (1982).
11 Stratmann, W.C.: A demonstration of PROMIS: the problem oriented medical information system at the Medical Center Hospital of Vermont, NCHSR Research Summary Series. DHEW Publication No. (PHS) 79–3247 (National Center for Health Services Research, Hyattsville 1979).
12 Weed, L.L.: Medical records, medical education, and patient care (Year Book, Chicago 1970).
13 Young, E.M.; Brian, E.W.; Hardy, D.R. (eds): Automated hospital information systems workbook (University of California Center for Health Services Research, Los Angeles 1981).

J.L. Lichtenstein, MD, Fourth St. and Highland Avenue, Lewistown, PA 17044 (USA)

Front. gastrointest. Res., vol. 7, pp. 46–65 (Karger, Basel 1984)

SYLVICS: A New System of Computerised Clinical Records

Claude Jeanty

Hôpital d'Ixelles, Service de Médecine (Dr. *A. Delcourt*), Bruxelles, Belgium

Introduction

How can computer science assist in the management of clinical records? A fundamental distinction should be made between the assessment of the patient management and the assessment of the clinical record. If some useful questions or investigations are omitted, or if some useless investigations are performed, these omissions or abuses should not be imputed to the record itself. Of course the better the patient management, the more interesting the clinical record. But the primary objective of the clinical record is to make the access to the existing information, whether appropriate or not, as easy as possible.

After discharge of the patient, his conventional record is put aside. If a physician wishes to restudy it and compare it with a hundred similar cases, the tedious task is frequently performed manually. If the patient is later readmitted, the record is scanned. The thicker the record, the more superficial the scanning. Usually only the discharge summary is carefully read.

A computer can serve both objectives: clinical research and patient care.

To demonstrate how chaos can become structure, how a data cemetery can become a data base, the factual information contained in the clinical record of an actual patient named Mike Allison will be traced along its journey through SYLVICS*[1].

[1] Each word followed by an asterisk is defined in the lexicon at the end of this chapter.

The Computer Input: the Relevant Information

Mike Allison, a 73-year-old retired constable, was admitted on the 9th September 1981 for haematemesis and melaena. He was pale, his pulse rate was 100, his blood pressure 110/70. An emergency endoscopic examination, by the author, demonstrated that in the superior portion of the duodenum there was a large and deep ulcer with a severe surrounding inflammation. The haemoglobin was 11 g/dl. The patient received 1,200 mg of cimetidine intravenously per day during the first 2 days and 1,000 mg orally per day thereafter. He was also given a transfusion of 3 units of blood, he improved quickly and could be discharged after 1 week. Such is the relevant factual information.

Two days after admission his clinical record was already 20 pages thick, cluttered with such statements as: 'mild tendency to chronic constipation', 'sluggish digestion of fatty food' or, among the progress notes, 'a second gastroscopy is arranged for next Tuesday', and so on. This kind of trivial information is not worth being stored in a computer. If the physician in charge of the patient would agree to put aside the factual information of permanent interest, the source paper record would become immediately ready for computer input.

The Translation

For the sake of confidentiality, Mike Allison's record will be identified only by the following number: 9080721 001 71. The first group of numbers, called in the retrieval program *birth**, provides Mike Allison's date of birth. The second group, called *sex**, indicates that Mike Allison is a male. The third group, called *check**, is simply a checking number.

The main fact [9] to be introduced into the computer is *haematemesis*. This is a compound term formed from two Greek roots: *haima, haimatos* = blood and *emesis* = vomiting. Yet SNOMED* contains only pure semantic primary terms. Therefore, if *haematemesis* is looked for in its alphabetic index, the reader will be referred to *haemorrhage* and *vomitus*. Whereas *haemorrhage* is regarded by a clinician as a symptom, it is considered by a pathologist as a morphological finding. So its SNOMED code begins with the letter M. *Vomitus* is a topographic term. Therefore, its SNOMED code begins with a T. So *haematemesis* will be introduced into the computer as M37000 and T6Y300. The link* of the first word*, which is its seventh and last character and links it to the following word, will be the letter I put for the preposition *in*. Thus, the whole phrase*, that is the smallest information entity, becomes more readable for the physician: *haematemesis* is translated into *haemorrhage in vomitus*. Though derived from a single Greek word: *melaina* = black, the symptom *melaena* will have a similar construction: *haemorrhage in faeces* coded M37000I T6Y100b (b represents a blank character). But in this case, to distinguish between upper and lower gastro-intestinal bleeding, a semantic modifier* must be added. *Black* could have been chosen. *Old* has been judged more specific. This being a subjective option, it is necessary to keep a dictionary of such options, in order to speak a universal language.

In SYLVICS, every phrase is determined by two or three coordinates*: section (Functional, Morphological or Laboratory data), date, and an optional coordinate diagnosis. As the information concerning the upper gastro-intestinal haemorrhage was collected from the patient through history-taking, it will be classed among the *Functional data*. Therefore, its section coordinate will be F, despite its belonging to the SNOMED *Morphology* axis*. As the haemorrhage occurred on the 9th September in 1981, the date coordinate will be 9810909. And as this haemorrhage belongs to the first diagnostic subset* of data that is considered, the diagnostic coordinate will be the first letter of the alphabet A. A first quartet*, that is a phrase and its three coordinates, is thus completed. The whole record will then be processed in the same way.

On admission, still on the 9/9/1981, the complete physical examination revealed nothing but pallor, tachycardia and hypotension. The next quartet will contain a one word phrase, *complete physical examination*, coded P023101, whose axis is P for *Procedure*, duodecimal code* is 02310 and link is 1. This digit 1 orders the computer to print the next phrase, which is also the next line, with one indentation for better readability. The section coordinate will be M, since a physical examination is classed among the *Morphological data* of the computerised record. The date coordinate is again 9810909. There is no diagnostic coordinate since the procedure *physical examination* brings no factual information by itself. The fact is *pallor*, quite logically coded as a *Morphology* word M04090b and printed, as already mentioned, with one indentation, as follows:

Complete Physical Examination

Pallor

The coordinates of the phrase *pallor* are M, 9810909 and A. Indeed *pallor* obviously belongs to the same diagnostic subset as *haemorrhage*, already labelled A. *Tachycardia* and *hypotension* could have followed *pallor* in the same phrase. But as precise numbers are usually available, this data is better included among *Numerical data*, where two specific columns are reserved for pulse rate and blood pressure, two *Function* terms. Thus, this quartet will be coded F71920b N100bbb F70600b N11/7bb and its coordinates will be N, 9810909 and A. The letter N means in each case *Numerical*, in the first case *Numerical* axis, in the second case *Numerical data* section coordinate.

An Endoscopy Report

Mike Allison's physical examination was followed by an upper digestive tract endoscopy. As this happened to be performed by the author, the endoscopy report contained no unnecessary comments such as 'the mucosa of the gastric corpus has a normal colour, there is no hiatus hernia, the pylorus is easily passed through', etc. As the oesophagus was normal, it was simply qualified as 'normal'. And so was the stomach. But the superior part of the duodenum was fully described as follows: 'anterior ulcer of 12mm, deep with necrosis, stenosis, congestion and oedema'. Such a description is ready for immediate coding, because it is a noun phrase. Most descriptions written in so-called free or natural language would contain verbs and would not allow easy translation and retrieval. In the above description, the word sequence is formalised as follows: site, colon; location adjective(s); main lesion, other adjectives; satellite lesions, linked by the preposition *with*.

The whole endoscopy report is thus printed in five phrases or lines. First phrase, the title *endoscopy*, coded P130001, a *Procedure* word, whose axis is therefore P, and whose link is 1, ordering one indentation for the next line.

The second phrase concerns the first organ observed: *oesophagus*: *normal*. A *Topography* word, T62000:, whose axis is T and whose link, a colon, announces that the following word(s) will describe the findings concerning that topographic location. Then a *Morphology* word, M001001, whose axis is M and whose link, 1, orders again one indentation for the next line.

Third phrase: *stomach: normal*, coded T63000: M001001.

Fourth phrase: *duodenum*, coded T643002. The link, 2, orders a further indentation for the following phrase, meaning that it will concern a sublocation of the duodenum, in this case its superior portion. The mention of the term *duodenum* implies that the whole duodenum has been seen through the endoscope. If only its superior portion had been examined, the comprehensive location, duodenum, would have been omitted. Thanks to this rule, the reader, as well as the computer, is informed about the sites which have actually been investigated during any procedure, without it being necessary to list all sublocations found normal.

The fifth and last phrase is reproduced exactly like the original, being coded as follows:

duodenal
superior
portion   *ulcer* *of* *12*   *mm* *, deep*   *necrosis*   *, congestion*
T64400: S17030b M38000V N12bbbb S31103, S16550W M54000, M34100, M36100A M36500b
   : anterior   *with*   *, stenosis*   *and edema*

This last phrase is the only phrase in the endoscopy report which gives factual positive information. Furthermore, this information is of major interest since it gives the main diagnosis of Mike Allison's record: *duodenal ulcer*. Of course the diagnostic coordinate of this last phrase will be the same letter A as for the haemorrhage and the pallor. These three elements form a diagnostic subset which now has a name *duodenal ulcer*.

The Versatility of the Curriculum vitae

All diagnoses or disease names are gathered in a special section of the computerised record: the *Curriculum vitae*, which constitutes the table of contents of the record. If the clinician just wants to glance at the patient's medical history, he will find a summary of it in the *Curriculum vitae*. So the phrase *duodenal ulcer*, this time not as a procedure finding but as a diagnosis, will be inserted into the *Curriculum vitae*. Therefore, its section coordinate will be C. Its diagnostic coordinate is of course A. But what is its date coordinate? Neither the date of the haemorrhage, nor the date of the endoscopy. The only appropriate date in such a chronic disease is the date of its first manifestation, 1965, which was quite simply collected by the history-taking.

The *Curriculum vitae* is not a mere list of diagnoses. It also turned out to be the right place to record the causes and treatments of diseases. Indeed a single a etiology, such as alcoholism, may be the cause of several diseases.

Furthermore, a disease or a treatment may be the cause of another disease. All these relationships can be indicated by inserting the diagnostic coordinate of the influenced diagnosis next to the factor that plays a causal rôle, whether a known aetiology, another disease or a treatment.

In Mike Allison's case, after a single painful episode in 1965, his duodenal ulcer disease had remained latent. Why this relapse after 16 years? Mike Allison had been a constable. He was retired, but despite a degenerative arthropathy of his right hip joint, he continued to tend his kitchen-garden and to ride his bicycle. Such was his peaceful way of life. On the 19th June 1981, 3 months before his haematemesis, he was run over by a car, resulting in a fracture of his right ankle. This important information will be coded as follows:

fracture *victim, cyclist, traffic accident*
Phrase: M12000V TY9510, FY3840b
of right ankle,
Section coordinate: C
Date coordinate: 9810619
Diagnostic coordinate: B

After a few weeks, Mike Allison became depressed, for he realised that it would be a long time before he could resume his usual way of life. Moreover, his bicycle was badly damaged and the insurance company was not hurrying to compensate him. He lost his appetite and some weight and, under those circumstances, his old duodenal ulcer reactivated. It is easy to emphasise these relationships in the *Curriculum vitae* by inserting the right diagnostic coordinates in the right places. Here is an excerpt of Mike Allison's *Curriculum vitae* showing, on the right of the dates, the proper coordinates of each diagnosis, and on the left of the dates, the coordinates of the influenced diagnoses:

	1965	*A*	*Duodenal ulcer*
	1976	*C*	*Degenerative arthropathy*
D	*19. 6. 1981*	*B*	*Fracture of right ankle, victim, cyclist, traffic accident*
A	*7. 1981*	*D*	*Psychological depression*

The letter D on the *fracture* line indicates that this trauma was the cause of his depressive state. The letter A on the *depression* line means that this stress influenced the subsequent evolution of the ulcer disease.

As to the coding of Mike Allison's treatment, there is no particular problem. Here is the continuation of its *Curriculum vitae* with some corresponding codes (the default dose unit is mg per day):

		E82070b P12X00b N1200bD N2bbbbb S12030b
9. 9. 1981	*A*	*Cimetidine intravenous injection 1200 during 2 days*
11. 9. 1981	*A*	*Cimetidine 1000 during 6 weeks*
12. 9. 1981	*A*	*Blood cell preparation 3 units in 2 days*
		E84330b N3bbbbb S30000I N2bbbbb S12030b

Laboratory Data

Laboratory data are frequently computerised at their the source. The problem is the transfer from one computer to another. In SYLVICS pattern, specific columns are designed and labelled for the 78 commonest analyses, allowing to print 328 results on one page, together with their equivalent in a universal scale [8]. This scale provides a quantitative assessment of the severity of an abnormality, for higher values as well as for lower values. For instance 600 indicates a marked increase, whether it concerns the blood sugar, the bilirubin, the transaminases or any other parameter. 40 indicates a severe decrease, whether for red blood cells, prothrombin, serum albumin, or anything else. The normal results range from 100 to 199. The universal equivalent of Mike Allison's admission haemoglobin (11 mg/dl) is 83.

Coding

The laboratory data will not be taken into account since it will be automatically transferred from the laboratory computer to the main computer. As for the other data, two methods will be compared: automated and so-called manual encoding.

When encoding is automated, terms as such are typed on a keyboard and afterwards they are converted into codes by the computer itself. The spelling of each term must be strictly respected. Of course the language is not free: only the terms belonging to the thesaurus may be used. The main advantage of automated encoding is its speed. Its main disadvantage is the cost of programming and of thesaurus storing.

In the alternative manual method, terms must be typed in the form of codes. It is cheaper, but tedious, stress-inducing and somewhat slower. However, the input speed can be increased by preselecting the terms which are most commonly used. Besides it should be emphasized that codes have, on average, half the number of characters of the corresponding terms. To give an extreme example, FY3840 is the code of *victim, cyclist, traffic accident*. Therefore, though the typing of code characters which do not mean anything is slightly slower than the typing of term characters which are comprehensible, the typing of a code is quicker than the typing of the corresponding term.

As far as frequency of use is concerned, terms can be classified into three levels. On the first level are the terms which are systematically used in a specific topic, such as upper gastrointestinal bleeding. They amount to less than 1% of the whole nomenclature. They can be displayed on a single large sheet of paper, in the same pattern as the computerised record. Moreover, most of these few hundreds of terms can be easily memorised. A second level is a gastroenterological microglossary* containing 2,300 terms, i.e. less than 5% of the entire nomenclature. The third level is the SNOMED itself.

In a trial assessment, 89 terms out of 100 were found in the first level list, 9 were found in the microglossary and only 2 required a search in SNOMED. Fortunately, under these practical conditions the encoding time becomes quite similar to the typing time. This similarity allows the dictating of the codes on a simple tape recorder and subsequently listening to the recording and typing at the same speed, without continuously having to switch the recorder on and off. A test, comparing both methods with the same clinical record, yielded the following results:

Typing time for 100 terms:	26 min	coding time for 100 terms:	19 min
		Typing time for 100 codes:	19 min
Total input time:	26 min	Total input time:	38 min

Most clinical records dealing with upper gastrointestinal bleeding did not exceed 100 terms, laboratory data excluded. It may therefore be concluded that, with the manual method in this specific topic, the total input time per record will usually not exceed 40 min. This total input time should be compared with the time required for dictating and typing a conventional discharge summary. It should also be pointed out that most of that input task can be assumed by paramedics.

I. M. C. IXELLES
MEDECINE INTERNE
908072100171

DATE: 08 OCT 1982

CURRICULUM VITAE

	1965	A	DUODENAL ULCER
	1976	C	DEGENERATIVE ARTHROPATHY
D	19. 6.1981	B	FRACTURE OF RIGHT ANKLE, VICTIM, CYCLIST, VEHICULAR OR TRAFFIC ACCIDENT
A	7.1981	D	PSYCHIC DEPRIVATION
	9. 9.1981	A	CIMETIDINE INTRAVENOUS INJECTION 1200 DURING 2 DAYS
	11. 9.1981	A	CIMETIDINE 1000 DURING 6 WEEKS
	12. 9.1981	A	BLOOD CELL PREPARATION 3 UNITS IN 2 DAYS

I. M. C. IXELLES
MEDECINE INTERNE
908072100171

DATE: 08 OCT 1982

FUNCTIONAL DATA

7.1981	D	ANOREXIA
	D	BODY WEIGHT LOSS 0.04 IN 2 MONTHS
9. 9.1981	A	HEMORRHAGE IN VOMITUS
	A	HEMORRHAGE IN FECES, OLD DURING 1 DAY

I. M. C. IXELLES
MEDECINE INTERNE
908072100171

DATE: 08 OCT 1982

MORPHOLOGICAL DATA

9. 9.1981		COMPLETE PHYSICAL EXAMINATION
	A	PALLOR
		DIGITAL EXPLORATION PER ANUS
	A	FECES: HEMORRHAGE, OLD
		PROSTATE: INCREASE IN SIZE
		ENDOSCOPY
		ESOPHAGUS: NORMAL
		STOMACH: NORMAL
		DUODENUM
	A	DUODENAL SUPERIOR PORTION: ANTERIOR ULCER OF 12 MM, DEEP WITH NECROSIS, STENOSIS, CONGESTION AND EDEMA
		RADIOGRAPHY OF THORAX
		ALL BRONCHI: SLIGHT SCLEROSIS
		JOINT OF THORACIC VERTEBRA: OSTEOARTHRITIS
		RADIOGRAPHY OF ABDOMEN
	C	HIP JOINT, RIGHT: OSTEOARTHRITIS
17. 9.1981		ENDOSCOPY
		ESOPHAGUS: NORMAL
		STOMACH: NORMAL
		DUODENUM
		DUODENAL SUPERIOR PORTION: ANTERIOR ULCER OF 8 MM WITH MODERATE STENOSIS, EDEMA, CONGESTION
26.10.1981		ENDOSCOPY
		ESOPHAGUS: NORMAL
		STOMACH: NORMAL
		DUODENUM
		DUODENAL SUPERIOR PORTION: MODERATE STENOSIS, A FEW EXUDATES

Appendix 1.

The Computer Output: the Polyptich

A new type of clinical record [7] for individual patient care, with the sophisticated structure previously described, comes out of the computer, a CDC Cyber 170/750, through a Pascal program. 3 pages of Mike Allison's computerised record, excluding the laboratory data, are reproduced in Appendix 1. This record will be continued, hand-written, until the next computer updating.

The Computer Core: the Data Base

The main interest of SYLVICS is still its data base, which is expected to answer any question about its contents. This last stage of the system is still under development.

At present, in a preliminary stage, a single typing of the data on an Apple II Plus microcomputer creates two files. One file is sent to the CDC computer to construct the data base. The other one is a sequential file, simply organised in quartets, to be managed through the microcomputer. This will test the capabilities of the conceptual structure, independent of the technical data base structure.

The data base is structured as a network according to the Codasyl recommendations and to the various constraints described above [6]. In summary, a clinical record is identified either by its serial number or by the patient's identification number. A clinical record contains a series of paragraphs*. A paragraph is identified by the record number and by its own serial number. It includes a date coordinate and a section coordinate. It is related to one or several phrases. Each phrase is identified by the record number, the paragraph number and by its own serial number. It occasionally includes a diagnostic coordinate or a causal relationship letter. It is related to one or several words. Each word is identified by the record number, the paragraph number, the phrase number and by its own serial number. It includes a SNOMED code and a link character and is related to the SNOMED thesaurus.

Training on a Microcomputer

40 simple sequential files have already been queried through the Apple computer itself. In the hope of assisting the prognosis of patients admitted for upper gastrointestinal bleeding, the following 9 questions have been asked: (1) Age? (2) Diagnosis? (3) Concurrent congestive heart failure?

(4) Previous ischaemic heart disease? (5) Previous respiratory failure? (6) Previous renal insufficiency? (7) Previous hepatic insufficiency? (8) Admission haemoglobin? (9) Active haemorrhage seen at endoscopy?

Several recent articles have emphasised the influence of the age, the clinical context and the presence of a visible vessel on the outcome [3, 5, 11, 12].

These 9 questions can be regarded as 9 variables, which can have, all together, 38 values. Variables 3–7 and 9 can each have only 2 values: present or absent. The age is classified into 9 classes. Seven diagnoses are considered: duodenal ulcer, gastric ulcer, hiatus hernia, erosive gastritis, Mallory-Weiss syndrome, oesophageal varices and other. Haemoglobin values are classified into 10 classes: 3, 4, 5 . . . up to 12 g/dl or more.

When a non-professional program written in Pascal was applied to Mike Allison's file, the program variable *birth* was assigned the value 9080721. The program variable *start* was assigned the value 9810909. The variable *age* which has the value *start* minus *birth* became 730188. In the program, if *age* is less than 800000, then the variable V1, that is the answer to the first question, becomes 70–79 years.

As far as the diagnosis is concerned, the algorithm is a little more complicated. If the section coordinate is F (*Functional data) and* if the first term of the phrase is M37000 (haemorrhage) *and* if the second term is T6Y300 (vomitus) *or* if the second term is T6Y100 (faeces) *and* if the third term is S11410 (old), then a new variable called *disease* is assigned the value of the corresponding diagnostic coordinate, in Mike Allison's case the letter A. In the next stage, if the section coordinate is C (*Curriculum vitae*) and if the date coordinate is less than or equal to *start and* if the diagnostic coordinate equals *disease* (in this case A) *and* if the axis of the first term equals D (*Disease* axis of SNOMED), then the program procedure *diagnosis* is activated. That procedure tells the computer that if the first term of the relevant phrase is D61041, then the variable V2, that is the answer to the second question, becomes *duodenal ulcer*, which was indeed Mike Allison's diagnosis.

In Mike Allison's record, the answer to questions 3–7 and 9 were *negative* and the answer to question 8 was 11 g/dl. No doubt the algorithms will be much simpler when the CDC data base is used.

This series of 40 clinical records, though very short, has a distribution of diagnoses and outcomes similar to that found in the literature [10, 11], that is:

Peptic ulcer	45 %	Good outcome	82.5%
Hiatus hernia	20 %	Bad outcome	17.5%
Erosive gastritis	7.5%		
Mallory-Weiss syndrome	7.5%		
Oesophageal varices	7.5%		
Other	12.5%		

A good outcome with conservative management was labelled 'Call a physician'. A survival due to an operation, or a death, was labelled 'Call a surgeon or a priest'.

The Probable Outcome of an Upper Gastrointestinal Bleeding

As the Bayes' formula was programmed in the microcomputer, caution was taken that the variables were not dependent and that the values were mutually exclusive and sufficiently discriminating.

As to the first condition, if the 9 selected variables are not totally independent, they are at least not closely related. Clearly, most patients with bleeding oesophageal varices had hepatic insufficiency, but several cirrhotics did not bleed from oesophageal varices. Renal insufficiency was linked to old age, but most aged patients kept a perfect renal function. Mallory-Weiss syndromes and erosive gastritis patients were all related to an admission haemoglobin greater than 12, but the same value was observed with many other diagnoses.

As to the second condition, even in cases of multiple lesions, there was always a single cause for the haemorrhage, so the seven different values of the variable *diagnosis* are actually mutually exclusive in this respect.

As to the third condition, the likelihood ratio between the two outcomes amounts to a minimum of 2 for at least one value of each variable (except for ischaemic heart disease). For example, an admission haemoglobin greater than 12 was 5 times more frequent among the good outcome group than among the bad outcome group. Appendix 2 shows the two series of 38 likelihoods which have been used in Bayes' formula. The following are the most discriminating values in decreasing order of power:

Predictive for good outcome	Predictive for bad outcome
haemoglobin 12 or more	haemoglobin 7
duodenal ulcer	renal insufficiency
age 60–69	hepatic insufficiency
	age 90 or more
	congestive heart failure
	oesophageal varices
	visible bleeding vessel
	respiratory insufficiency

Appendix 2. Likelihoods of each of the 38 possible values of the 9 selected variables, with respect to both outcomes

Variable	Value	Likelihood, %	
		in good outcome	in bad outcome
Age	0–19	0.1	0.1
	20–29	0.1	4.8
	30–39	6.1	4.8
	40–49	6.1	4.8
	50–59	18.2	9.5
	60–69	30.3	9.5
	70–79	18.2	9.5
	80–89	18.2	28.6
	90 or more	3.0	28.6
Diagnosis	duodenal ulcer	18.2	28.6
	gastric ulcer	27.3	14.3
	hiatus hernia	21.2	14.3
	erosive gastritis	9.1	0.1
	Mallory-Weiss	9.1	0.1
	oesophageal varices	6.1	14.3
	other	9.1	28.6
Congestive heart failure	presence	6.1	14.3
	absence	93.9	85.7
Ischaemic heart disease	presence	12.1	14.3
	absence	87.9	85.7
Respiratory failure	presence	24.2	42.8
	absence	75.8	57.2
Renal insufficiency	presence	3.0	28.6
	absence	97.0	71.4
Hepatic insufficiency	presence	12.1	42.8
	absence	87.9	57.2

Appendix 2. Continued

Variable	Value	Likelihood, % in good outcome	Likelihood, % in bad outcome
Admission haemoglobin	3 g/dl	0.1	0.1
	4 g/dl	0.1	0.1
	5 g/dl	8.0	0.1
	6 g/dl	8.0	14.3
	7 g/dl	8.0	42.8
	8 g/dl	8.0	9.6
	9 g/dl	8.6	9.6
	10 g/dl	8.6	9.6
	11 g/dl	8.6	7.2
	12 g/dl or more	41.9	7.2
Active haemorrhage at endoscopy	presence	21.2	42.8
	absence	78.8	57.2

Appendix 3 shows the computed posterior probability for each of the 40 patients to have a good outcome. Of course a 2% probability to have a good outcome is equivalent to a 98% probability to have a bad outcome.

It does not seem sensible to rely on a 50% discriminating level, since the prior probability for a good outcome is already 82.5%. This means that an unknown patient has a priori an 82.5% probability to have a good outcome. With an intermediate cut-off point at 61%, the computer predictive accuracy is 95%. Indeed only 2 good outcome patients are then wrongly predicted and are therefore expected to be overcared for, which is presumably harmless. With a cut-off point at 23%, the computer accuracy is also 95%. But in that case, 2 bad outcome patients have an overoptimistic prediction and the surgeon or the priest might be called too late. Whatever the cut-off point between 23 and 61 % the computer accuracy does not go lower than 92.5%.

Finally, since scepticism is the first step towards wisdom, two surprising findings. Firstly, the computer accuracy has been retested without the variable *diagnosis*. The accuracy remained 95%! Secondly, a simple scor-

Appendix 3. Posterior probabilities of good outcome

	100%	ooooooooooooo
	–	ooo ooo
	–	ooo
	–	ooo
	–	
	90%	
	–	
	–	
Prior probability	–	
	–	o
	80%	
	–	o o
	–	
	–	
	–	
'Call physician'	70%	o
	–	
	–	
	–	o
Best cut-off point	–	o
	60%	x
	–	
	–	
	–	o

o represents a patient who had a good outcome.
x represents a patient who had a bad outcome.

Appendix 3. (Continued)

'Call surgeon/priest'	–	x
	50%	
	–	
	–	
	–	
	–	
	40%	
	–	
	–	
	–	
	–	
	30%	
	–	
	–	
	–	o
	–	x
	20%	x
	–	x
	–	
	–	
	–	
	10%	
	–	
	–	
	–	x
	–	x
	0%	

o represents a patient who had a good outcome.
x represents a patient who had a bad outcome.

ing system, based on likelihood ratios, requiring no computer, already applied by the OMGE Research Committee to the diagnosis of inflammatory bowel disease [1], has also been tested on the same 40 patients. It reached an accuracy of 92.5%!

Should it be concluded that neither diagnosis nor computer can be efficiently exploited in the management of clinical records? It is hoped that SYLVICS will convince the reader of the contrary.

Lexicon

Axis. The first letter of a word*, indicating the field to which it belongs. Also that field itself. There are seven SNOMED* axes: Topography, Morphology, Etiology, Function, Disease, Procedure, and Occupation, respectively identified by their initial letters: T, M, E, F, D, P, except J (Job) for Occupation. Two additional axes have been introduced in SYLVICS*: Number and Semantic modifier*. Example: the axis of the word M37000I is M for Morphology.

Birth. A numeric variable formed from the first seven digits of the identification number of a patient's record, corresponding to the inverted date of birth, allowing to compute the age of the patient at the time of any event. Example: the date of birth 21st July 1908 becomes *birth* 9080721.

Check. The number formed from the last two digits of the identification number of a patient's record. *Check* allows to check the accuracy of the input and is computed as 97 minus the remainder of the division of the number formed from the first 10 digits of the identification number by 97.

Coordinate. A clinical record is regarded as a 3-dimensional space, where each phrase* is determined by 3 coordinates. The abscissa is the section coordinate: C for Curriculum vitae, F for Functional data, M for Morphological data, and N for Numerical data (see also SYLVICS*). The ordinate is the date coordinate, written with seven digits as an inverted date (example: 9th September 1981 becomes date coordinate 9810909). The third coordinate is the diagnostic coordinate, indicated by a letter.

Diagnostic Subset. A set of several phrases*, scattered throughout the clinical record, but determined by the same diagnostic coordinate*. A diagnostic subset should usually have a name, mentioned in the *Curriculum vitae* (see also SYLVICS*). Example: the following three phrases from a diagnostic subset named *duodenal ulcer*:

Haemorrhage in vomitus
Pallor
Duodenal superior portion: anterior ulcer of 12mm

Duodecimal Code. The duodecimal number formed from the five medial characters of a word*. Each of these characters may be one of the 10 digits or X or Y. Examples: the duodecimal code of the word M37000I is 37000 (haemorrhage), the duodecimal code of the word T6Y100b is 6Y100 (faeces).

Link. The seventh and last character of a word* which links it to the following word. The link may be a letter, a digit or a punctuation mark. A letter is an abbreviation of a preposition, a conjunction or a participle, such as I for *in*, A for *and*, or R for *relieved by*. A digit orders the computer to print the following line with that number of indentations, each further indentation indicating a more internal location. Among punctuation marks, only the following are used so far: ()*:,‹›?/ with their usual meanings. When none of these functions is necessary, the link is a blank character, noted b in the text.

Microglossary. An excerpt from SNOMED* designed for a specific purpose, such as gastroenterology, surgery, forensic medicine.

Paragraph. A logical sequence of phrases* determined by the same section and date coordinates*, for example an endoscopy report. The different phrases of a paragraph, though related to each other in respect to medical practice, may belong to different diagnostic subsets*.

Phrase. The elementary information entity, constituted by a series of words*. Example: *Duodenum: ulcer. Ulcer* alone is not a phrase. If *duodenum* alone is used as a one-word phrase, it only means that the whole duodenum has been examined and it must be followed by one or several other phrases. Most phrases correspond to a single line in the patient's computerised record.

Quartet. A phrase* with its three coordinates*.

Semantic Modifier. An additional axis*, indentified by the letter S, introduced in SYLVICS* in order to enable a flexible translation of any detail contained in the source paper record. The semantic modifiers are essentially 300 adjectives (classified into aspect, chronology, colour, complication, consistency, degree and topography) and 30 unit identifiers.

Sex. A numeric variable formed from the three digits following *birth** in the identification number of a patient's record in order to distinguish patients who have the same date of birth. As soon as a patient is registered in the system, he or she is assigned a three-digit serial number, odd for males, even for females. Example: 001 following *birth* 9080721 is attributed to the first male patient who was born on the 21st July 1908 and is registered in the system. The third female patient born on that date would be assigned *sex* 006.

SNOMED. An acronym for *S*ystematized *No*menclature of *Med*icine, created by the College of American Pathologists [2]. Thanks to its three major qualities: completeness, multi-axial structure and numeric hierarchical structure, it becomes possible to encode the entire factual information of any clinical record. SNOMED contains 50,000 terms, classified into seven axes*: Topography, Morphology, Etiology, Function, Disease, Procedure and Occupation. Its numeric hierarchical structure has five digits corresponding, from left to right, to more and more specific concepts. This allows the input of generic as well as specific terms and thus enables sorting on either statistical clusters of data or on hyperspecific details [4]. The only important modification to SNOMED that had to be made in SYLVICS* is in the Digestive Disease nomenclature where 200 terms have been replaced by 500 terms, hierarchically classified. The only important addition is the new axis Semantic modifier*. This modification and this addition, together with some other additional terms concerning drugs, family members and countries form the SYLVICS addendum to SNOMED, copies of which are available from the author.

SYLVICS. An acronym for *Sy*stem of *l*ongitudinal and *v*ertical *i*nformation *c*oded in *S*NOMED*. This computerised system is essentially a data base formed from a set of highly structured clinical records. Each record is a subset of diagnoses, some of which, called diagnostic subsets*, are subsets of phrases*. These phrases, determined by two or three coordinates*, are classified into three sections: *Functional, Morphological* and *Laboratory* data. The diagnoses, together with their causes and treatments, are gathered in a fourth section called *Curriculum vitae*. Being written exclusively in key-words, this new clinical record is readable either by a clinician for individual patient care or by a computer for clinical research.

Word. Each seven-character element of a phrase*, constituted by an axis* (one letter), a duodecimal code* (five characters) and a link* (one character). Example: M37000I (haemorrhage in).

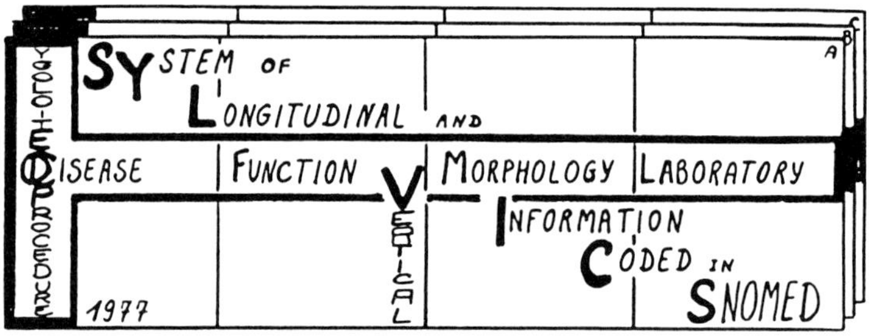

Acknowledgements

Profound gratitude is due to *Sylviane Jeanty* for her constant and invaluable cooperation in the field of encoding and thesaurus management, to *Patrick Isbendjian* for the design and implementation of the data base and for the editing program of the polyptich, and to *André* and *Yvette van Melsen* for their efficient help in programming.

References

1 Clamp, S.E.; Myren, J.; Bouchier, I.A.D.; Watkinson, G.; de Dombal, F.T.: Diagnosis of inflammatory bowel disease: an international multicentre scoring system. Br. med. J. *284*: 91–95 (1982).
2 College of American Pathologists: Systematized nomenclature of medicine; 2nd ed. (College of American Pathologists, Skokie 1979).
3 Conn, H.O.: To scope or not to scope. New Engl. J. Med. *304*: 967–969 (1981).
4 Côté, R.A.; Robboy, S.: Progress in medical information management: Systematized nomenclature of medicine (SNOMED). J. Am. med. Ass. *243*: 756–762 (1980).
5 Griffith, W.J.: The visible vessel as an indication of uncontrolled or recurrent gastrointestinal hemorrhage. New Engl. J. Med. *300*: 1411–1413 (1979).
6 Isbendjian, P.; Jeanty, C.; Machgeels, C.: A SNOMED coded data base for medical records; in Begon, Anderson, Saito, Walters, Côté, Yasaka, Proc. 2nd Annu. WAMI Meet., Versailles 1979, pp. 9–13.
7 Jeanty, C.: The computerised medical record in gastroenterology: an original design using SNOMED: in Shires, Wolf, Medinfo 77, pp. 283–287 (North-Holland, Amsterdam 1977).
8 Jeanty, C.: The computerised medical record in gastroenterology. 3. Numerical laboratory data. Med. Inform. *3*: 291–297 (1978).
9 Jeanty, C.; Jeanty, S.; Pajot, A.; Isbendjian, P.; Machgeels, C.: Problems of translation of free medical language into SNOMED: personal experience; in Velthoven, Proc. of the 8th Int. Congr. on Health Records, vol 1, pp. 67–76 (The Hague 1980).
10 McGinn, F.P.; Guyer, P.B.; Wilken, B.J.; Steer, H.W.: A prospective comparative trial between early endoscopy and radiology in acute upper gastrointestinal haemorrhage. Gut *16*: 707–713 (1975).
11 Morgan, A.G.; McAdam, W.A.F.; Walmsley, G.L.; Jessop, A.; Horrocks, J.C.; de Dombal, F.T.: Clinical findings, early endoscopy, and multivariate analysis in patients bleeding from the upper gastrointestinal tract. Br. med. J. *ii*: 237–240 (1977).
12 Storey, D.W.; Brown, S.G.; Swain, C.P.; Salmon, P.R.; Kirkham, J.S.; Northfield, T.C.: Endoscopic prediction of recurrent bleeding in peptic ulcers. New Engl. J. Med. *305*: 915–916 (1981).

Note Added in Proof

Following the preparation of this chapter, two improvements have been made. Through the use of mnemotechnic abbreviations, included in the input program, the total input time for 100 terms could be reduced to 25 minutes. The querying has now been performed on the CDC data base and, as expected, the algorithms are not fundamentally different, though the manipulation has become much quicker.

C. Jeanty, MD, Hôpital d'Ixelles, Service de Médecine (Dr. A. Delcourt),
B-1050 Bruxelles (Belgium)

Front. gastrointest. Res., vol. 7, pp. 66–95 (Karger, Basel 1984)

Data Management in a Gastroenterology Service Using a Microcomputer

M. Ward

Department of Gastroenterology, Royal Brisbane Hospital, Brisbane, Queensland, Australia

Introduction

The main objective of electronic data processing (EDP) is the conversion of related facts into useful information. Until recently this facility has only been available at a high cost and in a relatively inaccessible form, as the available computers were large, expensive and difficult to operate. They were therefore centralized and their use restricted to EDP professionals with specific training. The advent of the microcomputer, however, has widely increased the availability and drastically reduced the cost of computing. The large market base of video game players, programmable calculator users, and electronic enthusiasts has stimulated the development of increasingly sophisticated machines which cater for the 'small business' requirements. This has been possible as a result of the substantial increases in memory and processing power of microcomputers which have diminished the functional distinction between these machines and their larger counterparts. Software development has generally lagged behind that of hardware, but this is now being corrected as programs produced for large computers are modified and imitated with enthusiasm and ingenuity by both professionals and amateurs. The potential for microcomputers in clinical data processing is obvious, but there are limitations as well as advantages which need consideration.

The purpose of this chapter, therefore, is to attempt to answer three questions: (1) For which task can a computer be effectively used in clinical data storage and analysis? (2) How do the particular advantages and disadvantages of a microcomputer compare with those of a larger system? (3) What are the practical considerations in the design and implementation of a microcomputer system in a clinical unit?

Whilst the comments and descriptions which follow are derived from experience gained in the introduction of a microcomputer system in a department of gastroenterology, they could equally be applicable to the needs of many specialized units.

The Potential Value of Computers

Data Processing. Any specialist unit, or indeed any medical department, inevitably accumulates a large number of facts, mostly from contacts with a patient. Whilst specific requirements will vary from unit to unit, there will always be a central core of facts which will commonly need to be stored and collated for current and future use; these are listed in table I and are sequentially generated as a result of a single transaction arising from a request for information about a single patient. The essential data processing requirement is a transmission of the information about the pa-

Table I. Facts accumulated by specialist units

Facts related to	*Facts*
Identification	patient's name date of birth sex hospital number address, etc.
Origin	reason for referral source – private doctor – other hospital – other clinic/ward
Procedure or consultation	text report of procedure or consultation diagnosis drugs used treatment given complications staff identification
Future activity	check laboratory results further procedure clinic visit

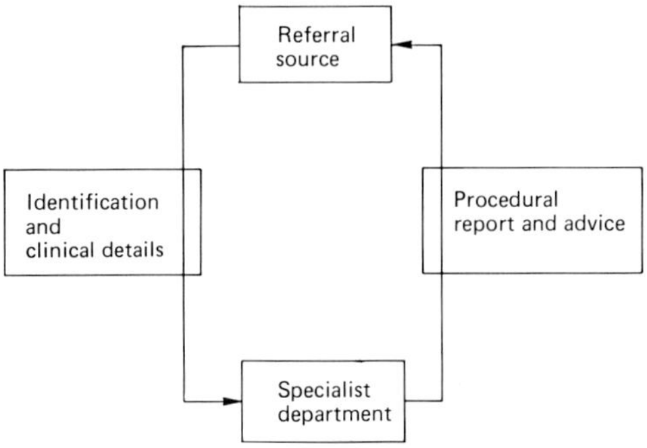

Fig. 1. Normal information flow.

tient between the referral source and the specialist department (fig. 1). Traditional paper forms or chart systems are usually developed which meet this requirement reasonably efficiently. EDP techniques have little to offer this transaction except possibly to speed up the transmission of information. Problem arise, however, when any other view of the information contained in this simple loop is required, or when the passage of time has degraded the capacity of the traditional recording methods to provide the original information. These additional views are essential components of efficient administration, quality control, and research. They require the juxtaposition of large numbers of related items of information to allow recognition of paterns of similarity, and to assess the influence of time on the occurrence of particular events.

It is in such functions that computers far exceed the capacity of paper records. Their ability to extract and analyse data in large groups helps overcome a natural human tendency to underestimate the inherent unreliability of small samples [14]. The information which needs to be extracted and the form in which it is presented will be determined by the level at which it is required (table II).

Typical questions for which large-scale views might provide answers would include: (1) How many patients with a given diagnosis come from a particular source? (2) What is the age and sex distribution of patients presenting with a particular system? (3) Is the work load of a particular procedure changing? (4) What is the complication or success rate for a procedure when performed by a particular physician? (5) Have all the subjects in a high risk category for certain diseases been adequately reviewed?

Table II. Levels and categories of information

Level	*Category*	*Example*
Hospital	strategic	cost/value estimates
Departmental	tactical	work load projections
	operational	procedural success rate
	individual	patient details

Table III. Will a computer solve the problem?

Yes if it requires	*No if*
Rapid storage and recall of data	problem is not clearly defined
Collation of like groups	data is disorganized
Comparison of different groups	system is not tailored to needs of the department
Rapid arithmetic	

These and many other questions can be answered by regrouping and re-examining the data once it is stored in the computer. Rapid extension of applications beyond those originally proposed commonly follows the introduction of a computer. However, it must be certain that the questions asked are answerable by a computer, and preliminary organization of the data with clear definition of the objectives is essential (table III). Also, the system must be adapted to the work of the unit and not vice versa. Publications extolling the virtues of medical computing must be interpreted with caution. There is often an unfortunate tendency for computer enthusiasts to be dazzled by displayers of technology. Their papers are written in the future tense, describing what a system can do, rather than what it has done. The road to computerization is not smooth. It has been estimated that only 20% of published medical computing projects were subsequently routinely used by their authors [7]. This high failure rate is probably due to the pursuit of objectives that were machine-determined rather than environment-determined, and to failure to take human-machine interactions into account [5, 16]. Elegant answers to unnecessary questions are of little help.

Other Functions. In addition to clinical data processing there are other facilities which are now available in both large and small computers which are attractive to specialist units.

(1) Filing. An obvious additional filing function for which computers could be used in medical units would be the storage and analysis of literature references. Whilst massive multiuser data base system such as Medline are now widely available, there remains a need for local collection of items of particular interest to the unit which can be accessed rapidly and cheaply [2, 10].

(2) Word Processing. Any physician who has had to correct and edit numerous drafts of scientific papers and submissions will appreciate the value of word processors. It makes little sense to purchase 'stand-alone' word processors if the same function is provided by a computer which can also perform many other tasks.

(3) Statistics. Numerous packages are now available which allow sophisticated analysis of data already stored by the computer. The computer is both more flexible than programmable calculators, and has the advantages of displaying data graphically which often eases interpretation.

(4) Teaching. Computer-aided instruction is now well established and software is available either in the form of specific multiple-choice questions or problem-solving sequences, or in packages which allow the development of such sequences by the teacher.

(5) Terminals. With the rapid growth of computer networking via telephone lines and an increasing number of large medical data bases becoming available, access to this massive store of information is a considerable bonus. This is now possible with most microcomputers.

Staffing Implications. In a commercial environment the motivation for computerization is clear – to increase profitability through increases in efficiency and reductions in the work-force. In specialist medical practice this is rarely the prime consideration. In most departments clerical staff are usually a small part of the work-force, both numerically and in salary costs compared with nursing, medical and paramedical components. Clerical staff are also usually multifunctional – they are responsible not only for filing/data analysis, but also function as typist, secretary, receptionist and telephonist. Thus, the labour-saving component of computerization will be accompanied by an increase in work in other areas, and by developments of new projects which the computer allows. The primary advantage of computerization in such units lies in the greater access to latent information already collected but not otherwise accessible, and in the increased efficiency of administrative and scientific functions. It is probably for this reason that computerization of private medical offices has not been as successful as might have been expected, other than in large group practices where accounting and billing capabilities justify the expense.

Microcomputer Possibilities and Alternatives

If it has been decided that a data processing problem exists which is solvable by a computer, the next decision concerns the type of system which is required – micro, mini, or large orthodox facility. The differences are essentially quantitative; the larger the system the greater the storage capacity and processing speeds. Inevitably more capacity costs more money, and financial resources are the usual final determinants of the system choice. As an EDP problem, the use of a computer for clinical data processing presents no novel difficulties. The requirements are very similar to those which have already been very adequately met for customer accounts, manufacturers inventories, insurance policy data, and many other commercial applications for many years. Thus if funds are available for access to a large machine and the necessary expertise, there is little point in turning to microcomputers. It should be stressed, however, that if an orthodox system is to be used, it is essential that it should have sufficient capacity and that the professional personnel who will control access, have the time and interest to evaluate the unit's problems, and to implement and maintain the solution. Unfortunately sometimes there is a communication problem between medical and EDP professionals, neither fully appreciating each others problems and limitations. Also, EDP departments in public hospitals are frequently understaffed and overworked for their primary administrative and financial responsibilities, and have little time to find solutions to the problems of individual clinicians and units.

There are two other factors which influence system choice. The first of these relates to capacity and processing speeds. Before the introduction of a computer into the department it is always difficult to estimate how much data storage capacity will be required. The usual tendency is to underestimate, but if the data processing needs are fairly orthodox and unspecialized, such as those outlined above, if it is acceptable to analyse data in groups of up to 1,000 cases at a time, and if speed of access is not critical, then the microcomputer is likely to be acceptable. Even if the ultimate storage requirements are of a size that will require large machine capacity, a microcomputer can still serve a very useful purpose as an initial evaluation system. This allows programes to be developed cheaply, exact requirements to be defined, and some data to be accumulated. When development is complete and storage capacity is exceeded, either the programs and data, or just the data, can be transferred to a larger computer with the microcomputer remaining as a terminal through which data can be entered and recalled. The need for even this conversion will probably disappear as very high capacity mass storage (hard disc) devices become available.

The second consideration is one of outlook of the physician concerned. If the computer is required as a 'black box' to perform a specific task, then large professional systems are probably most suitable. Alternatively, if there is an interest in mechanisms, and a desire to explore and exploit the full potential of the computer, then a microcomputer provides an ideal first contact. It is entirely self-contained within the department, without any external controlling forces, and is available for experimentation at leisure without any fear of embarrassment that novices sometimes feel when confronted with large computing systems with professional guardians.

There have been relatively few descriptions of microcomputer applications in clinical data processing, although there are publications relating to history recording [9], disease registers [11], and clinical audit [15]. Doubts have been expressed by professional managers as to the suitability of microcomputers for small group specialist practice for clinical data processing and accounting [6], but successful applications of this type have been described [13]. The professional reservations mostly concern memory size, system reliability, and the availability of appropriate software. The rate of development of both hardware and software will almost certainly ensure that these reservations are only transient.

Design and Implementation of a Microcomputer System

The essential stages of computerization, usually accomplished in sequence, are system analysis, hardware acquisition, software development and implementation. All four stages are recognized as essential for computerization in commercial environments but the first and last are in danger of neglect when microcomputers are used. This is in part due to the promotion of microcomputers by their vendors as 'instant' solutions to data processing problems.

Systems Analysis

Although this section is written using experience gained with a microcomputer, much of it is applicable to the introduction of any computer system. Systems analysis comprises the definition of the data processing load and the organization of the data in a form that can be efficiently processed to achieve the overall objectives. It is perhaps the most vital stage of the whole process of computerization. It is for this reason that systems analysis is a whole science in itself and a subdivision of the data processing industry. In commercial terms, the systems analysis needs of a specialist unit are relatively simple, but if professional assistance is available it should be used. The analysis will consist of a close examination of how the unit generates data and in particular *why*. The purpose of computerzation is not simply to produce an electronic copy of current paper practice but to achieve efficient storage of the minimum data required for the overall objectives. Paper record system often encourages the storage of excessive data which has little information value and which will hardly ever be used. This is probably because little thought has ever been given to *why* the facts are recorded, and because most humans feel more confident with large amounts of data, even if they know they are never likely to use it [4]. The storage of redundant data increases cost and slows access time. It is important that systems analysis should not be considered as a once only event, but as an integral and recurrent component of computerization which will have to be continued as the system develops and generates new requirements and exposes new areas of ignorance (fig. 2).

(1) Definitions. Any collection of related data has to be organized to three levels for efficient access (fig. 3). *The record* is the group of facts relating to the object of the data processing, in this case the patient, and contains all items relevant to that individual – name, age, sex etc. The *field* is the space occupied by the data items of a single type from one or more records. The *file* is the total collecton of all records which need to be analysed as a group. Records within a file may be stored *sequentially* and accessed via an index file or *randomly* and accessed via some predeter-

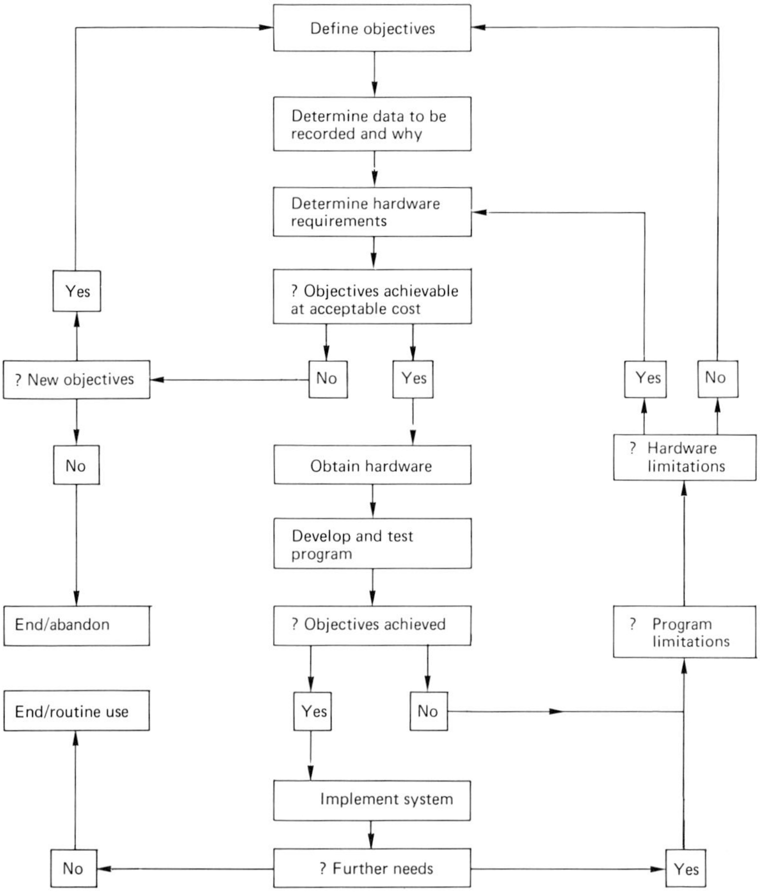

Fig. 2. The computerization process.

mined scheme such as alphabetical or numeric ordering. Records may be of either *fixed* or *variable* length. Fixed length records are usually simpler for programming purposes, but are neither so flexible nor so efficient in the use of storage space as variable length records.

Various specialized software methods have been developed to allow rapid access by a variety of routes to different components of groups of related data items. The inter-related data items are known as *data base systems* and the programmes controlling access to the data as *data base managers*.

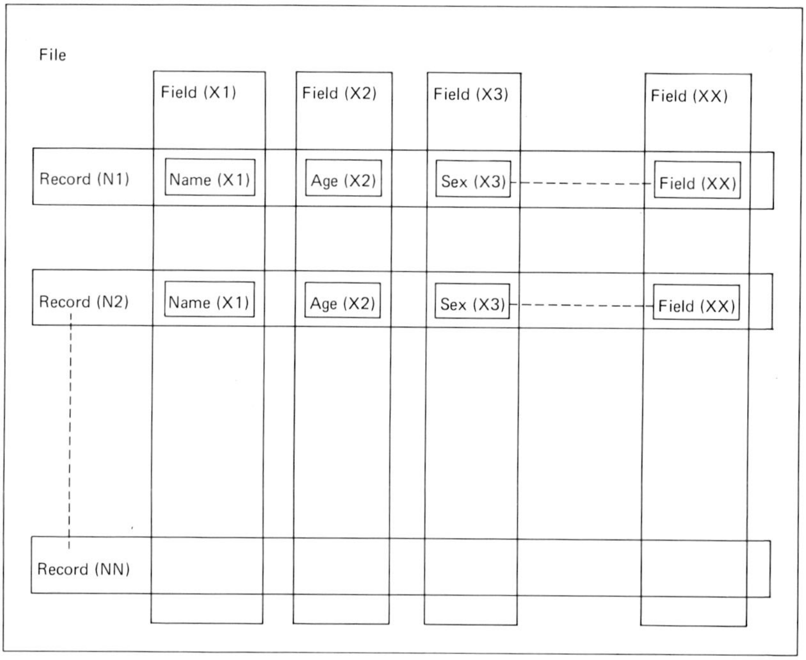

Fig. 3. Files, records and fields.

(2) System Analysis Requirements in a Department of Gastroenterology. Examples of the sort of information which may need to be gathered in a systems analysis in a department of gastroenterology are shown in table IV.

(a) Memory Capacity Estimates. Although much information can be coded and memory storage requirements thus decreased, some, such as text reports, cannot. It is therefore important to know not only the total number of patients but also the number of items to be recorded per patient and the length of the procedural reports. Estimates are made in numbers of characters, one character per letter, item of punctuation, or space. Generally 1 byte (a unit of memory space) is required for the storage of one character. A reasonably accurate estimate of the upper limit of storage space requirements for text reports may be obtained from the value given by the mean + 2 standard deviations of a sample. These estimates are particularly important if fixed length records are to be used, as input in excess of the allocated space will result in truncation and data loss. They are not

Table IV. Systems analysis in a department of gastroenterology

Surveyed	*Required for determination of*
Total number of various patient contacts	total memory storage space
Routine information recorded per patient	
Average procedural report lengths	
Special category usage	
Number of referral sources	coding arrangements
Number of indications for referral	
Number of procedures	
Number of diagnostic categories	
Number of patients requiring recall	
Frequency of access to files	mode of data storage
Speed of access to files	
Alphabetic distribution of patients' surnames	
Completeness of individual data items	validity of analysis

so critical if variable length records are used but are still required for calculations of the total number of records that it will be possible to store on a single disc.

(b) Coding. The use of coding can allow substantial reductions in storage space requirements. Numerical codes are generally easier to handle for program purposes than alphabetic. The total space required will depend upon the number of potential entries – up to 9, 1 space, up to 99, 2 spaces, up to 999, 3 spaces, etc. It is better to over-estimate than under-estimate, for example if the number of diagnostic categories currently in use is 80–90, then it is best to allow 3 digits to allow for the inevitable additional diagnostic categories that will be required to be added from time to time and which will increase the number of possibilities beyond 100. Increased numbers of coding possibilities can be achieved if necessary, but utilizing the computer's ability to examine for both likeness and position, and by adding the full range of keyboard characters to the usual numeric codes.

Thus, a 2-digit code using alphabetic and numeric characters could include A–Z and 0–9 in two positions, i.e. AA–ZZ or 00–99, or A0–Z9, etc. allowing a total of 1,296 codes compared with 99 for numeric codes alone. The essential requirement is to estimate the maximum likely number of different entries in each category. It is also useful to determine the most commonly encountered entry in a category, as it is a relatively simple matter to program for single-key stroke default entry. This provides considerable savings in typing times for frequently used data. It is also possible to provide automatic coding to save table look-up-time and to allow for entry of previously unencountered categories with subsequent allocation of new code numbers on review. Such facilities are worth the additional programming effort, as it is by its ability to handle exceptions and previously unencountered entries that success or failure of a system is frequently determined. If a scheduling function is to be incorporated it is obviously essential to know the maximum duration of follow-up and a rough estimate of the numbers of patients likely to be recalled, to allow construction of suitably sized files.

(c) Mode of Data Storage. If a system is to be used primarily for research purposes, the speed of access to individual items will not be critical, but if individual patient data is to be available immediately for telephone queries, etc., the construction of files must allow sufficiently rapid access. Such requests generally arise within 3–6 months of the procedure or consultation, and data accumulated during this time can usually be stored on one or two discs. It is therefore also important to know the frequency of requests and for how long these continue. Rapid access is achieved by several file or distribution methods; one of these, random access, is usually organized so that data is kept in alphabetical or semi-alphabetic order. If such a system is to be used, a preliminary analysis of alphabetic distribution of a sample of surnames of the local population will be required to ensure efficient utilization of disc space. Another and more commonly used system utilizes an index to allow rapid access to a sequential file, (indexed sequential access method, ISAM). Several different indices are possible, allowing different views of the data and different access routes.

(d) Validity of Analysis. Not much reliance can be placed on data for which more than 10–15% of potential entries are absent or invalid. It is therefore essential to determine that the facts which are to be recorded will be available in all or nearly all subjects and will be recorded in a form that can be easily coded and entered into the computer. Careful consideration of this issue and avoidance of any requirement to record data that is not agreed by all relevant staff to be essential will minimize negative entries. Doctors are notoriously unreliable data recorders. It is best to require them to record the minimum number of facts, and to leave actual data entry into the computer to clerical or other non-medical staff who are generally much more reliable for such work.

Hardware

There is now a confusing array of machinery confronting the potential buyer of a microcomputer system. Some of the factors which have a bearing on the choice are shown in table V.

Table V. Hardware choice factors

Central processor unit	memory size interface capacity upgrade potential
Video display unit	character/screen appearance
Permanent storage	floppy disc memory capacity double/single/density number of tracks number of slides access time hard disc memory capacity backup facilities operating system upgrade availability
Printer	upper/lower case 'letter quality' printing column width plotting/graphics potential
Software	operating system application programs data base managers word processors statistics
Others	service support other local users

(1) Central Processor Unit. This is the main core of the computer system and is usually housed beneath the keyboard. It contains two types of memory, the read-only memory (ROM) which carries the high level language (usually BASIC) and the random access memory (RAM) which is blank and available for programs and data. RAM size is critical, it is measured in thousands of bytes or kilobytes (KB). Little useful data processing can be performed with less than 32 and 48–64 KB is the more usual memory size. Machines are now coming onto the market, however, which can address memories in the region of 500 KB and which obviously offer enormous increases in computing power. Most machines currently used are based on 8-bit microprocessors. Whilst these are adequate, 16 bit-based systems are now appearing which will offer substantial advantages in processing speeds and power and in their ability to have several operators using the computer simultaneously. As with any very new machine, however, there will be a lag before adequate software is developed.

As the pace of development of microprocessor technology shows no sign of slowing, an important factor in the choice of any equipment is its potential for expansion to take advantage of additional facilities and memory capacity that are available now and those which will become available in the future. This is particularly important with regards to central processor unit (CPU), RAM and storage capacity, as program lengths and storage requirements usually increase when systems become operational. Discovery that the machine chosen has limited expansion capabilities is frustrating. Another feature which is now almost standard but is important is the capacity to link with other systems. It is usually achieved via an electronic interface and telephone connection device known as a modem. This facility not only provides access to vast information stores, but also to practically unlimited additional memory space for data storage on a rental basis. In summary, present capacity and potential for expansion are the prime considerations.

(2) Video Display Unit. Superficially all video display units (VDUs) appear similar but after several hours of work, the ease of use and avoidance of eye strain provided by some become apparent and important. Character size, colour, freedom from flicker, etc., should be checked if the VDU is to be heavily used. Direct inspection of the alternatives is again the best guide.

(3) Permanent Storage. Data and programs have to be stored in some permanent or semipermanent form. This is usually provided either by

'floppy' discs or increasingly by hard disc systems. Cassette storage is the cheapest option but is too slow and cumbersome for anything other than the most elementary functions. Most personal microcomputers utilize 5.25-inch discs but 8-inch discs provide greater capacity and there is some pressure to make these the industry standard. Capacity is not solely a function of disc size, features such as double-density and double-sided access can produce marked increases in capacity. This means that a single disc can store anything from 80 to 560 KB or more, according to type and size. Translated into record numbers and assuming that the average requirement per patient is about 250 bytes or 0.25 KB, the patient capacity per disc will vary between 300 and 2,000. Obviously, if this information can be coded and the number of bytes allocated per patient can be accordingly reduced, there will be substantial increases in the number of patient units of information that can be stored per disc.

Hard disc systems are now available for many microcomputers. These are usually fixed and raise the storage capacity of a single unit considerably. The smallest is usually in the 5-megabyte range. Using the same assumptions given above, this would provide immediate access to almost 20,000 patients. At present, these units are approximately the same cost as that of the computer itself – $4,000–6,000 – but the advantages are obvious.

Software and operating system compatibility have to be considered, however, if hard discs are to be added to an existing system and backup facilities must also be considered. The latter function is important as the prospect of an electromechanical failure destroying the records of 20,000 patients is obviously not attractive. Backup is usually provided by copying records onto floppy discs or tapes.

(4) Printer. These are essential to any serious computer installation, and there are now many excellent machines on the market at very reasonable prices – $500–2,500. If 'letter quality' printing for word processing is required, 'daisy wheel' type printers or their equivalent are essential and cost more than conventional computer-style printers. Graphics and plotting capabilities may be required and the total work load that the machine will encounter also needs to be considered. Small cheap printers, as well as being slower than the more expensive counterparts, also withstand prolonged heavy-duty office use only poorly.

(5) Software Availability. An important factor which may be concealed behind the impressive technological credentials of the latest

machine is software compatability. This applies both to operating systems and to high-level languages.

(a) Operating Systems. These are the programs, usually loaded from disc at power-up, which control the transport of data between CPU and disc and which organize the distribution of data on the disc. They are usually written in machine language. Each manufacturer usually produces a specific version for their own machine, e.g. TRSDOS for TRS 80, APPLEDOS for Apple, etc. Others, such as NEWDOS and DOSPLUS, are produced by independent operators and frequently have additional features which facilitate programming and operation. CP/M is another operating system now widely used and may become an industry standard, and this would have considerable advantages in terms of program exchange. CP/M compatability in a machine is therefore an advantage and allows access to many professional programs. On the other hand, the larger manufacturers, such as Tandy and Apple, which have been in the market for longer periods, have accumulated large numbers of programs utilizing their own operating systems.

(b) High-Level Languages. The above remarks apply to high-level languages. All manufacturers supply BASIC but dialects vary, and rewriting programs for different machines is tedious. Many business programs are written in COBOL and scientific programs in FORTRAN and these are also offered by most manufacturers.

(6) Other Factors. Maintenance and local support are important considerations. Here again, the larger organization such as Tandy and Apple have the advantage of extensive networks of local suppliers and maintenance organizations to help with inevitable electromechanical faults that occur. In this context, the presence of other users of a particular machine in the locality can be of considerable support, both for hardware and software problems as they arise.

Application Software Development

This section will deal with the development of programs for clinical data processing, and will exclude consideration of programming for any of the other functions outlined above. As with any enterprise, professional systems will probably provide the best solution in the shortest time, and

Table VI. Software-to-hardware cost ratios

	1950s	*1960s*	*1970s*	*1980s*
Hardware, %	70	35	20	15
Software, %	30	65	80	85

programming is no exception. However, the cost may be considerable. The ratio of software to hardware costs has changed progressively in favour of hardware over the past 20 years (table VI) [3]. A few months of professional programming assistance costs several thousand dollars and very soon exceeds the hardware costs. There may also be the additional expense of recalling programmers to correct any problems which may, and frequently do, arise in the first year or so of use, or for any additional requirements that may become apparent. In general, therefore, there is little point in combining low cost microcomputers with high cost professional programming unless there are very specialized requirements. The choice is between commercially available packages and owner-user programming.

(1) Pre-Packaged or Customized? When affordable computing first became a reality, successful use was entirely dependent upon the availability of programming skill. This is no longer the case. Several commercial packages are now available which allow data to be stored easily and which provide powerful analytic possibilities. These data base managers (DBM) have been produced for most popular computers at very reasonable prices – $ 100–500. Observation of the use of such packages in several specialist departments in a teaching hospital suggests that they will be satisfactory for the majority of clinical data processing needs. Whether they will be satisfactory in an individual case depends on both personal considerations and general requirements.

(a) Personal Considerations. Although amateur programmers can produce flexible and valuable programs which are well adapted to the particular needs of a department and which are produced without the direct cost of professional assistance, this solution is by no means universally applicable. Programming is arduous and time-consuming, and although some find it pleasurable and stimulating, to others it is a tiresome and incomprehensible chore. Some are so fascinated by the intrinsic logic and

Table VII. Essential features of data storage systems

1	Controlled input format
2	Storage organized for ready access
3	Ability to alter or delete data
4	Ability to search for individual data items or groups of related items
5	Ability to organize related items in a particular order, e.g. alphabetic
6	Ability to present data in a useful way – printouts of items found or sorted

mechanisms of the microcomputer and enjoy the intellectual stimulation that practical programs rarely emerge. At the opposite extreme the 'clinical realists' are only interested in the outcome of what the computer can do for them. They care little of how this is achieved and should avoid trying to develop programming skills. The message is clear – the best programs are produced by the pragmatists who find the middle way – they are sufficiently interested in mechanisms to overcome the frustrations of programming while keeping firmly in touch with the overall requirements of a system that will have to work in a real clinical environment.

If there is no spontaneous attraction to programming it should not be forced out of fear of missing the oft-described 'microelectronic revolution'. Whilst microcomputers are currently maximally exploited by those with programming skills, this will change as commercial software is developed which performs commonly required functions in a way that is largely invisible to the non-programming user. Indeed, the revolution will not reach its peak until such software is developed and the larger market that this brings is exploited. For most applications, use of a microcomputer will then be no more dependent on programming skill than enjoyment of music played on a cassette recorder is currently dependent on the ability to compose or perform music.

(b) General Requirements of Data Storage Systems. The essential features of a data storage system, whether ready made or specifically written, are shown in table VII. Data that is entered via the keyboard must be subject to predetermined checks of character type and number to ensure validity of subsequent analysis. Data must be organized so that it can be both stored and recalled rapidly and there must be facilities to alter data before and after storage. It must be possible to search for related items, to organize these items in a particular way or order, and to present this information either to the VDU screen or to the printer. These bare essentials are provided by all commercially available data base managers to a greater or lesser degree. The more sophisticated DBMs provide many functions in addition, some of which are described below. This approach is a commercial necessity reflecting the need to accommodate as many different environments and requirements as possible, but is not without its disadvantages. In smaller capacity microcomputers, either free data space in the CPU is sacrificed, or multiple disc input-output operations slow access time, as separate program segments are loaded. An otherwise excellent system will be of no use if it contains many features that are not required at the expense of many that are. For example, some DBMs have fixed length fields restricted to 40 or so characters which may present difficulties if larger entries of text are required.

All particular requirements can be provided by specifically written programs, and the choice between package and tailored programs may be difficult if the personal considerations mentioned above do not exclude one approach or the other. The simplest solution is probably to obtain a data base management system and try it. This will add little to the cost of the hardware and even if it does not prove suitable for the main clinical data processing function, many other uses will inevitably be found – references, specific studies of small groups of patients, etc. Also, experience with such a package is often a valuable means of further defining and refining the exact requirements of the department.

(2) Specific Features of DBMs. How is an appropriate data base manager selected? The best approach is to try to find a local user who has experience of the DBM in question on a similar machine, or failing this, to at least see it demonstrated by a local vendor or agent. It will generally be apparent whether it has the required capabilities, but some of the features which are worth special consideration are shown in table VIII.

(a) System Compatability. Most DBMs have been produced for a specific machine, although a few are produced in several versions for different machines. Whilst it is possible to operate some DBMs with a single disc drive, two are normally required. Software compatability with standard word processor and statistical packages is valuable. Storage capacity field

Table VIII. Specific Features of Data Base Management Systems

System compatability	hardware – CPU/disc drives/printer software – word processing/statistics
Storage capacity	record and field size total number of records per file disc drive span of files
Ease of use	documentation comprehensibility of screen display security of data provision for backup copies modification potential/language type
Input	errors traps field length restrictions cursor control field types alphabetic numeric calculated date default entry subsequent field addition potential correction pre- and post-storage audit trails
Search	relational operators single or multiple field instring/masked speed
Sort	ascending/descending speed single or multiple field store sorted file
Calculation	range of operators +/–/x/ etc. subtotals on listings
Printouts	columnar labels store print format

lengths are usually restricted and have to be specified during initialization, although some allow variable length fields. Total permissible record length (usually somewhere between 255 and 4,000 bytes), total number of records per file and whether a file can span more than one disc should also be considered.

(b) Ease of Use and Flexibility. This will be dependent upon a number of factors, especially documentation and programming design. Direct inspection of instruction documents and program demonstrations are the only sure way of assessment. If there is any desire to modify the program it must be ascertained that this is possible. Many DBMs are written at least in part in machine language, or may have inbuilt copyright protection, and are accordingly difficult or impossible to modify. If security of data is important for confidentiality, then this would require password protection. Dependence on magnetic material storage of important data demands consideration of copying or backup facilities.

(c) Data Input Controls. Input of data should be possible in alphabetic or numeric form. Better DBMs also allow specific data entry, single-key default for commonly used entries, calculated fields and cursor screen-position control for rapid entry and correction. Correction of both immediate and stored items should be easy, and global changes of all entries of the same type is a useful, if slightly hazardous facility. Data validity should be protected by input error traps. It should not be possible for example to enter alphabetic characters into a numeric field or vice versa. Two other valuable functions are the ability to add extra fields after the system has been used for some time and an audit trial feature which allows visual display of recent additions or changes.

(d) Search Functions. The critical function of any data processing system is its ability to rapidly extract the required information. It should be possible to search more than one field and to offer a full range of relational operators (and/or, less than/greater than, equals /not equals). For example, it should be possible to extract all patients of one sex less than a certain age with one diagnosis but not another. Good DBMs should be able to extract the required information from several hundred records in a few seconds. Whilst 'perfect match' searches for a field are invariably provided, the additional ability to search for a subcomponent of a field is extremely valuable. This may be of two types: the 'instring search' and the 'masked

Result of search for:

Name	Sm	Smith	Smythe	Smithson
S m i t h	+	+	–	–
S m y t h e	+	–	+	–
S m i t h s o n	+	+	–	+

Fig. 4. Instring functions – illustrating 'near match' and alternative spelling search possibilities.

Field position	1	2	3	4	5	6	7	8	Search result
Record 1	1	1	A	7	Z	2	6	J	–
2	A	7	X	2	Z	6	Z	Z	–
3	X	X	J	2	A	7	2	J	+
	Masked				Search window		Masked		

Fig. 5. Masked search functions – for codes A7 at character positions 5 and 6 with all other characters masked.

search'. The instring (searching '*in*' a '*string*' of characters) retrieves all records whose specified search-field contains the required character or group of characters anywhere in the field. This is useful in searching for near matches of names (fig. 4). A masked search is similar but allows both the component and its position in the field to be specified. This provides a vast increase in the amount of information which can be coded and stored in a single field (fig. 5).

(e) Sort Functions. Data frequently needs to be listed in order – typically an alphabetic listing of names or a list of biochemical values in decreasing order. All DBMs provide a sorting function but some are slow, either because the sort program is inappropriately written in a high level language rather than machine code, or because many inefficient disc input-output operations are required. Ideally it should be possible to rapidly sort more than one field at once, either in ascending or descending order and to be able to store the data in sorted form.

(f) Calculations. Automatic calculated fields are provided by the better DBMs. A field is provided with a formula and the machine calculates the required result from values given in other fields, e.g. field (A) = 32 units, field (B) = 8 units; field (C) = 10 units; field (D) = (A/B) × C = 40.

Such DBMs also generally allow column totals or subtotals to be derived when groups are searched for or printed, plus various other calculated functions. Linkage to more sophisticated packages to allow standard deviations, t-tests, regressions, and other statistical comparisions is often possible and a useful additional capacity.

(g) Printout. Hard copy of material that has been extracted and sorted should be available, at least in columnar form with columns (= fields) determined by the user and the display format organized as required. Most DBMs also provide a label type format and some allow form letters to be produced and for the storage of specified printout formats, so that instructions do not have to be given each time material is printed.

(h) Selection of Alternatives. In a rapidly developing and competitive market, final choice is often difficult. Computer magazines, such as 80 Microcomputing, Byte and Creative Computing, often feature comparative reviews of data base management and other software packages and are a useful source of information. Examples of just a few current DBMs that are in fairly wide use are shown in table IX.

(3) Customized Applications Programs. (a) Advantages and Disadvantages of BASIC. If commercial data base managers do not provide all that is required, then customized application programs have to be written.

Table IX. Available data base Managers

DBM	*Produced by*	*System*	*Approximate price, $*
D.B. Master	Stoneware	Apple	250
Maxi Manager	Adventure international	TRS 80	100
AIDS III	Meta technologists	TRS 80	100
Profile III Plus	Tandy	TRS 80	250

These will usually be written in the high-level language BASIC which is often dismissed by professional programmers as a slow and unsophisticated language. These criticisms may be valid but are largely irrelevant, and the fact remains that for low-cost computing BASIC has tremendous advantages. Not only is it widely available and easy to learn, but it is the language of thousands of application programs. Many of these are for filing functions similar to those required for clinical data processing. These are published in the many computer magazines and books that are now available or may be bought on discs at low cost. This provides the amateur programmer not only with material which can be modified for different filing functions, but also with examples which demonstrate how a particular objective is achieved.

(b) Modular Construction. The general objectives of data storage systems and of the desirable features of data base management systems have been described and are equally applicable to customized application programs. The objectives of the particular program should first be listed and subdivided into logical groups or units. The flow of information through these units should be traced and the impact of differing conditions and data determined. Time spent on this stage is well rewarded. Once the main modules in the program and their component parts have been defined, individual logical algorithms can be constructed and programmed. This modular approach shortens development time by allowing testing of individual units and correction of the inevitable logical and language errors before the modules are linked to provide the whole program.

Typical main program modules and their interconnections are shown in fig. 6. These interconnections are usually controlled by option lists or 'menus' which display the possible choices and direct control to the chosen module or submenu. When the relevant function is accomplished, the program returns to the sub or main menu for further choices.

(c) Subroutines. Certain repetitive functions which may be required by more than one of the main modules are best performed by way of subroutines. Some typical examples are shown in table X.

(d) Utilities. Only a small percentage of programming time is spent writing code instructions – the majority is taken up by testing and removing errors and rewriting segments. This tedious process is made much easier if certain utility functions are available. These are mostly provided in the

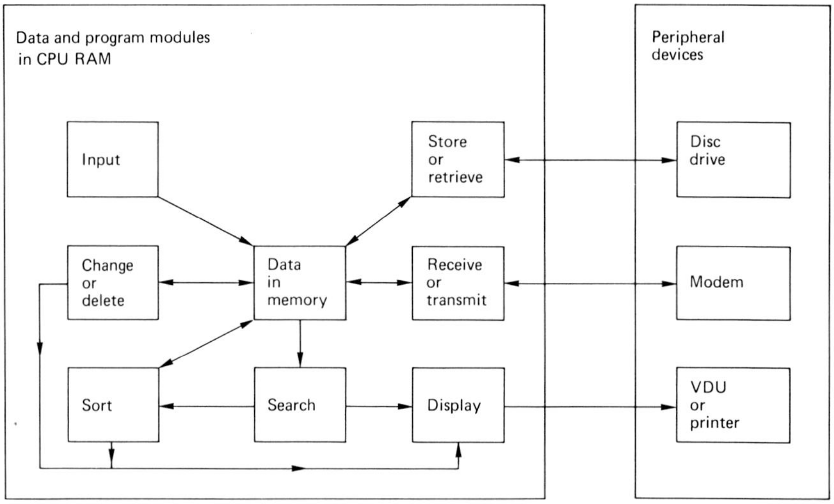

Fig. 6. Main program modules.

Table X. Typical subroutines

Messages	error warnings data input awaited operating advice
Print/display	column titles field/record contents
Calculations	means, ranges, etc.
Printer status check	
File handling functions	
Alphanumeric data range control	

operating system but may also be obtained separately on disc, or typed in from published listings. They consist of short programs, often in machine code, which provide functions such as line renumbering, line duplication, merging of program segments, active and passive variable analysis, and memory block moves. These functions are increasingly provided as standard features of operating systems and considerably facilitate programming. The general direction of software development is to allow the programmer more time to concentrate on the logic of the program design, thus relieving him of the work of organizing the control of the computer and its peripheral devices [1].

(e) Speed Enhancements. BASIC is a slow running language because of its structure and because it is usually provided as an 'interpreter'. This means that it translates each program line in sequence and passes on the instruction in machine code. Other high-level languages intended for larger machines, such as Cobol, are frequently provided with a 'compiler' rather than an interpreter. The program, once perfected, is translated in its entirety to machine code in which form it is then stored. Compiled programs run substantially faster than those which have to be interpreted. Some BASIC compilers are now available but are not widely used.

An alternative, and entirely acceptable approach, is to concentrate effort to increase speed on those modules which benefit from machine language, such as search and sort functions. Other parts of the program such as data input/correction and menu displays, do not usually repay the effort of machine coding, as BASIC is fast enough for such purposes and the response time is faster than most typists can enter data. For memory block moves, data searches and sorts, however, BASIC may require from several minutes to an hour or more to accomplish tasks which machine code can achieve in a few seconds. Machine code programming is hard and more time-consuming than high-level language programming and requires the use of special utility programs – editors/assemblers and monitors. Fortunately, there are several techniques of installing short modes of machine code in a BASIC program without full knowledge of machine language programming. Details of how to achieve such hybrid programming functions are available in books which also provide other valuable information for improving the efficiency and style of BASIC programs [8, 12].

(4) Implementation. It is a mistake to imagine that once a machine is obtained and software provided, the process of computerization is complete. Many months of testing in the real environment of clinical work and with non-expert operators will be required to uncover the inevitable procedural, logical and language errors and to match the system to clinical reality. The system should be stressed with as wide a variety of data input as possible in an attempt to uncover shortcomings. It should gradually be introduced in parallel with the paper system it will replace and there should

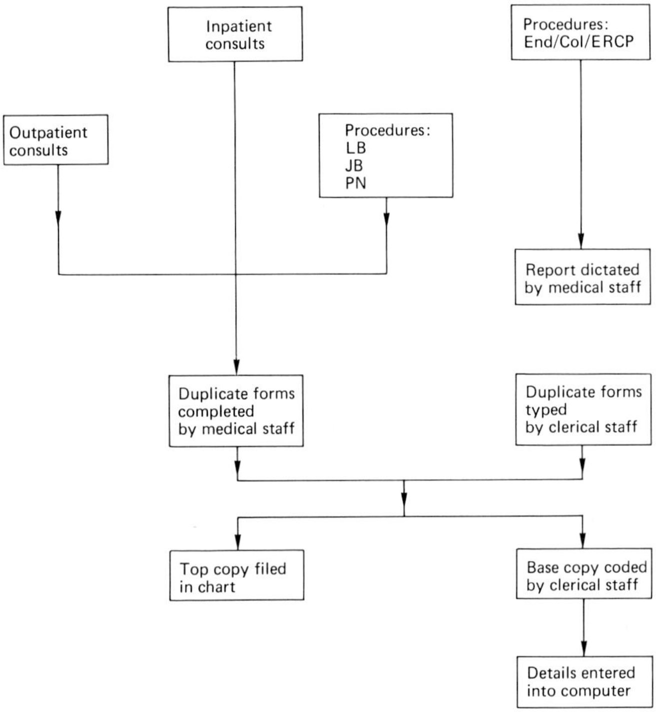

Fig. 7. Royal Brisbane Hospital, Department of Gastroenterology System – data input. End = Upper endoscopy; Col = colonoscopy; ERCP = endoscopic retrograde cholangiopancreatography; LB = liver biopsy; JB = jejunal biopsy; PN = parenteral nutrition.

be complete confidence in the new before the old is completely discarded. With implementation the essential question changes from why the process of computerization is necessary to how effectively the system performs in answering the question, and how it might be further refined, modified and developed.

An Example of a Working System

For the past 3 years the Department of Gastroenterology, Royal Brisbane Hospital, has used a microcomputer for clinical data storage analysis. The routes by which data is entered into the computer is shown in figure 7, the range of retrieval options in figure 8, and the storage space allocation in table XI. The hardware comprises a Tandy TRS 80 Model 3, 48 KB RAM

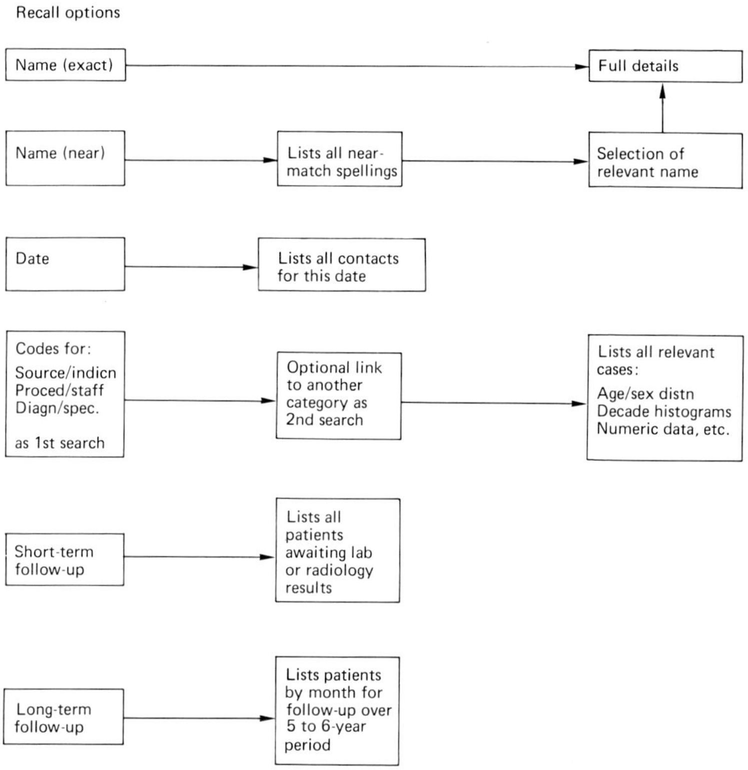

Fig. 8. Royal Brisbane Hospital, Department of Gastroenterology System – data retrieval.

CPU with two disc drives and a line printer. The main applications program has been written in BASIC by the author but commercial word processing, data base managers and statistic packages are also used. The system has proved reliable and has been well accepted and utilized. Its main uses has been in the extraction of diagnostic and procedural categories for clinical research and audit, and for the calculation and projection of work loads for administration [15]. Its main current limitation is its inability to store full text reports of endoscopic and other procedures. Acquisition of extra disc storage capacity and rewriting of programs is currently in progress and should overcome this limitation, allowing paper records to be discarded completely. Although the programs were developed for a specific unit and may thus be partially individualized, it should be possible to modify them for other similar gastro-instestinal units.

Table XI. Royal Brisbane Hospital, Department of Gastroenterology System – details stored per patient with byte or character space allocation

		Bytes			Bytes
1	Name	23	8	Staff	1
2	Hospital No.	6	9	Procedure	1
3	DOB	6	10	Diagnosis	9
4	Sex	1	11	Follow-up	6
5	Date of contact	6	12	Serial number	4
6	Referral source	2	13	Special	18
7	Indication	2		Total	85

Conclusions

Microcomputers can be used successfully for clinical data processing provided: (1) their current limitations of memory and speed are recognized and taken into consideration when applications are devised; (2) that there is careful prior definition of the purposes for which the data is to be processed and the methods by which it will be collected and organized; (3) that a machine with appropriate capacity is selected; (4) that the pre-eminent importance of relevant applications programs is appreciated: pre-packaged data base managers may be suitable if needs are fairly orthodox, but customized applications will fully utilize the power of the microcomputer; (5) that it is appreciated that the development of customized applications software by professionals is expensive, with costs that will probably exceed those of hardware; (6) that amateur programming is only successful where interest, enthusiasm and time are available.

It is probable that further dramatic increases in computing power and memory storage capacity will occur and will make microcomputers increasingly competitive with their larger counterparts. These developments, combined with the likely evolution of applications software for non-programming users, will provide powerful data processing ability for clinical units that have not previously enjoyed such facilities.

References

1 Bacon, G.: Software Sci. *215*: 775–779 (1982).
2 Bertrand, D.; Bader, C.R.: Storage and retrieval of bibliographic references using a microprocessor system. Int. J. bio-med. Comput. *11*: 285–293 (1980).
3 Branscomb, L.M.: Electronics and computers: an overview Science *215*: 755–760 (1982).
4 Davis, G.B.: Management information systems: conceptual foundations, structure and development, pp. 72–73 (McGraw-Hill/Kogakusha, Tokyo 1974).
5 Fox, J.: Development of hospital computing. J. R. Soc. Med. *72*: 425–431 (1979).
6 Freamo, B.E.; Landry, M.G.: Do microcomputers have a place in medical practice? Can. med. Ass. J. *122*: 706–707 (1980).
7 Friedman, R.B.; Gustafson, D.H.: Computers in clinical medicine. A critical review. Comput. Biomed. Res. *10*: 199–204 (1977).
8 Gratzer, G.A.; Gratzer, T.G.: Fast BASIC (Wiley, New York 1982).
9 Lilford, R.J.; Chard, T.: Microcomputers in antenatal care: a feasability study on the booking interview. Br. med. J. *283*: 533–536 (1981).
10 McCabe, J.B.; McCabe, B.H.: Microcomputer-based filing systems for emergency medicine literature. Annls Emerg. Med. *10*: 87–90 (1981).
11 Meldrum, D.: Simple computerised disease register. Br. med. J. *282*: 191–198 (1981).
12 Rosenfelder, L.: Basic faster and better (I.J.G. Inc., Apland 1981).
13 Trobridge, G.F.: Use of a microcomputer in a three physician practice. Can. med. Ass J. *119*: 770–772, 811 (1978).
14 Tversky, A.; Kahneman, D.: Belief in the law of small numbers. Psychol. Bull. *76*: 105–110 (1971).
15 Ward, M.: Microcomputer data storage and analysis for clinical audit. Aust. clin. Rev. *3*: 16–21 (1981).
16 Whitehouse, C.R.: Preparing to introduce a computer into a health centre. Br. med. J. *283*: 107–110 (1981).

M. Ward, MB, FRCP (Edin.), FRACP, Director, Department of Gastroenterology, Royal Brisbane Hospital, Brisbane, Queensland (Australia)

Front. gastrointest. Res., vol. 7, pp. 96–109 (Karger, Basel 1984)

Data Management in a Gastroenterology Endoscopy Service: Initial Experience Using a Minicomputer

P. Rozen[a], *E. Levy*[b]

[a]Municipal-Governmental Medical Center and Sackler Medical School, [b]Eddy Levy Scientific and Commercial Programming Company, Tel Aviv, Israel

Introduction

Some three decades have passed since computer services entered the field of medicine [8]. These services are used to analyze large amounts of data such as research projects and, more recently, to provide 'on-line' services for the storage, retrieval and immediate analysis of clinical information, a natural extension of this being to aid in decision-making [3, 7]. Parallel to the development of these programs ('software') has been the improvement in the equipment ('hardware') produced. Computers have become smaller physically, less sensitive to environmental changes, faster in their manipulations and cheaper to produce.

This has led to a change in computer philosophy, away from providing large, expensive 'mainframes' servicing a multitude of users, to providing small but powerful minicomputers for individual users, each with dedicated programs for his own particular need. The large computer, if available, is free for large projects, but can also be used as a data base for the minicomputer which in turn, may also function as one of its terminals.

For unclear reasons, gastroenterologists have lagged behind in utilizing computer technology [10]; in contrast, cardiologists rapidly introduced computer techniques to aid them utilize the technological changes in the catheter laboratories and intensive care units, by providing rapid data management and analysis.

The main technological advances in gastroenterology (GI) have been in the field of endoscopy. With the rapid introduction of various fiberoptic instruments during the last decade, many GI services are performing numerous diagnostic and therapeutic procedures. However, they are not efficiently utilizing the vast amounts of data – which are often being inadequately recorded and not easily available for retrieval. Because retrieval of patient information is difficult, gastroenterologists are not deriving the scientific benefit expected from their 'data-bank'; a bank of information which would naturally be the basis for diagnostic and decision analysis, analysis of cost-benefit for GI procedures, prognostic evaluation, etc.

Ab initio, better data management is needed. Since much GI data is generated through the endoscopy services, it is logical to begin there. Others have already tried this, namely *Kanzler* et al. [4] and *Frühmorgen* [2] in Germany, *Dobrönte* et al. [1] in Hungary, *Stalnikowitz* [11] in Israel, and *Pancotto* et al. [6] in the USA. However, all these are off-line systems that are inherently cumbersome, needing coding or a special work sheet and, therefore, wasteful of staff time, liable to errors, and dependent on the personal interest of the program initiator. To the best of our knowledge, most of the above system are not in active use. Recently, *Ward* [13] in Australia has described the successful use of an off-line microcomputer for data storage and analysis of endoscopy procedures and clinic visits. In this chapter, we will briefly review our experience in developing data management programs utilizing a minicomputer.

Requirements of the Computer System

In order to be useful, where possible the system should be on-line, thus 'paperless', avoiding the use of intermediate forms. It should be based on easily read, easily understood, and commonly accepted terminology, requiring a minimum of technological understanding and dexterity from the physician. The data entry should be as complete as possible, but in order to avoid a cumbersome format, may require separate and/or special management using free text. The advantages and disadvantages of a computer service and favorable characteristics required are listed in table I. Most are self-evident and will not be discussed further.

Aims of the Computer System

The computer programs needed by most GI units for data management are listed in table II. Obviously, the most commonly used programs

Table I. The advantages, disadvantages and characteristics required of a computer service

Advantages	*Characteristics*
Data storage on a large scale	low cost
Uniformity	modular and expandable
Fast and accurate data retrieval and analysis	multiple users possible
Data-bank for future use	small, no special housing or cooling
Aid to instrument management and patient follow-up	common languages available
Reduces use of office manpower	on line
	simple terminology
	easy retrieval
Diasadvantages	easy to read print-out
One time cost of software and hardware	versatile, not dedicated
Personnel need training	
Rigidity of format and language	

Table II. Computer programs needed for a GI unit

A. (1) Upper GI endoscopy	B. (1) Gastric ulcer follow-up
(2) Colonoscopy	(2) Colon polyp follow-up
(3) ERCP	(3) Ulcerative colitis follow-up
(4) Laparoscopy	(4) Screening for colorectal cancer
(5) Esophageal manometry	
C. GI Laboratory procedures:	D. Instrument control program
(1) Absorption test	
(2) Gastrin, CEA measurements	
(3) Other research programs, e.g. gallstone dissolution program	E. Word processing

will be for upper and lower gastrointestinal endoscopy. From these, subprograms can be derived for gastric ulcer, colon polyp follow-up [5] and even a screening program for colorectal cancer [9]. A further subprogram concerns instrument control. This is needed to follow the purchase, use and repair of the multitude of instruments commonly found in the modern endoscopy service.

The data entry should be direct into the computer terminal, integrating data entry with an immediate 'dialogue' with the computer, data verification, error checking, editing and response to enquiries. When needed a computer-derived report should be available immediately for verification and documentation. Safeguards are needed to prevent illegal access and for guarding of patient's secrecy. In our system individual passwords are given to each user. This allows limited access to the computer files. Only authorized and senior personnel are given passwords which enable overall entry to the computer data bank. Logical checks must be built into the system to prevent illogical data entry and the leaving out of essential information. This can be done by predetermining limits for measurements, and deciding what is the minimal information needed and the logical sequence of data entry. A mistake results in the error being indicated on the screen and this blocks further data entry until corrected.

Provision is needed for updating and correcting data; e.g. pathology results are received after the endoscopy procedure and occasionally may not confirm the macroscopic diagnosis. However, once data entry is completed by inserting the name of the authorized examiner, no corrections are allowed. Corrections and additional information are given as a supplemental report. This prevents possible legal consequences of the misuse of computer files. Basic statistical programs are required to allow the immediate derivation of simple data, such as total number, demographic data, listing of diagnoses, accuracy, etc.

Choice of Hardware

The choice of hardware depends on needs, budget and existing equipment available. The individual gastroenterologist working mainly in private practice, with minimal demands for data entry and memory, may well manage with a micro, 'personal', computer. However, a large GI department, with direct access to an institutional – 'mainframe' – computer, may find it simpler to join their peripherals by cable or by point to point (telephone) connection, to this computer. The advantages are obvious and include a rapid response and virtually unlimited data storage. The disadvantages might include the expense of being on-line, and dependency on other department's services. (The other department may have different priorities, over which there is little control).

The minicomputers available satisfactorily answer the computer needs for most medium-to-large GI units. The distributed data processing (DDP) system of these computers allows the department to be independent in their clinical and scientific work. These computers are relatively inexpensive and modular, allowing further additions according to developing needs. They allow many peripherals such as terminals and printers to work at the same time in parallel – while the excess memory and storage capacity can be shared by cable and so reduce costs. Physically, the units are not large, being the size of an ice-chest or small refrigerator; they work at average room temperature and do not require any special electrical fittings.

The memory of the processor units range from 64 KB to the powerful and fast 512 KB unit. We believe that 128 or 256 KB is needed for a medium to large GI unit. The external data storage disks range from 10 to 200 MB. The latter is preferable in order to maintain as much information as possible on-line. Diskettes, floppy disks or a diskette magazine, are useful for moving off-line, old or rarely used data. The modular nature of these computers allows future changes to be made, increasing the memory and storage capacity, and even allowing the unit to act as a terminal for a large computer. The terminals needed include at least one with a keyboard for both programming and data entry, and others with a simpler keyboard for just data entry. The printer chosen need not be fast, as output in a GI unit is not large, but the print-out should be easily readable to be useful as a report. For this reason we recommend a unit that uses changeable plastic ('daisy') wheels and will produce a print-out similar to that of a good quality electronic typewriter on normal quarto-sized paper.

In our department we chose to use an IBM Series/I minicomputer with a 256 KB memory, 64 MB storage disk and a 27.8 MB diskette magazine, shared by cable with a neighboring department [12]. The printers used include a high-speed matrix and medium-speed Xerox 'Diablo' printer.

Choice of Software

Well-known, high-level languages such as Basic, Cobol, PL/1 and Fortran IV should be used for the programs. They are provided with many minicomputers and this allows for most programmers to prepare and change programs as needed. We have found it convenient to use Fortran and Cobol for most of the programs.

Data Entry

The software programs are based on a series of prepared options. Following the entry of patient information, name, address, age, etc. (fig. 1), there follows a series of menus which allows the choice of program (fig. 2),

```
                                            GASTRO PATIENT'S FILE(R)

***   P A T I E N T ' S   I N F O R M A T I O N   ***

PATIENT'S IDENTIFICATION NO. _______________

ADMITTANCE DATE:  DAY __   MONTH __   YEAR __

FAMILY NAME ____________________   FIRST NAME ______________

DATE OF BIRTH:   DAY __   MONTH __   YEAR __       SEX _ (M/F)

COUNTRY OF ORIGIN ___________      FATHER'S NAME _______________

ADDRESS:    CITY ______________   ST. ______________   NO. ____

            ZIP __________       STATE ___________ TEL. _________

                                                  E. L. COMPUTERS LTD.
```

Fig. 1. Example of patient information screen.

e.g. upper endoscopy (fig. 3). This can be done by the departmental secretary or an assistant. Thereafter, the cursor rapidly and automatically goes from option to option and only relevant positive information is entered by pressing the 'Y' (Yes) key or a number, when appropriate.

The clinical information screens are shown consecutively (fig. 4), and then those relevant to the preparation for the procedure – premedication, instrument used, etc. (fig. 5). There are 3 menus for X-ray and endoscopic findings in the upper GI tract, esophagus, stomach and duodenum. This allows the examiner to record at the level of the menu (by merely registering the findings) or rapidly choose the screens he will require to fill in detail, both for radiology and endoscopy findings (fig. 6). These screens for data entry are basically of similar format and based on 4 questions: site, size, amount, and state (fig. 7). When several findings are present, e.g. 2 gastric ulcers and the examiner wishes to describe each separately, then the same screen can be filled in twice (gastric ulcer 1 and gastric ulcer 2), and the findings kept separate.

The final screens summarize the findings and identify the examiners (fig. 8). The endoscopy report is immediately available. This includes the personal information of the patient, symptoms, description of radiology and endoscopy findings and opinion of the examiner. The pathology results are entered later, when available, and sent as a supplement with appropriate comments, if needed.

As most patients have, at the most, one or two abnormal endoscopic findings; data entry by the physician or trained assistant takes only 2–4 min of his time. Not more than dictating a report!

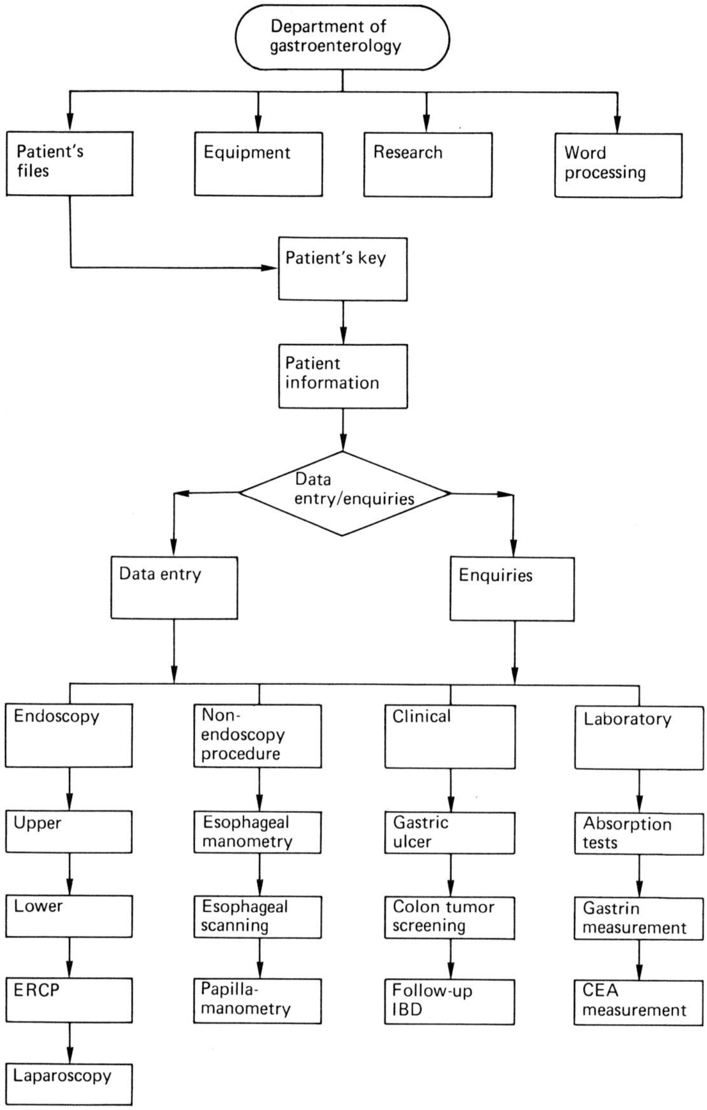

Fig. 2. Flow chart of patients' files allowing data entry, recall, updating and analysis through the various program alternatives.

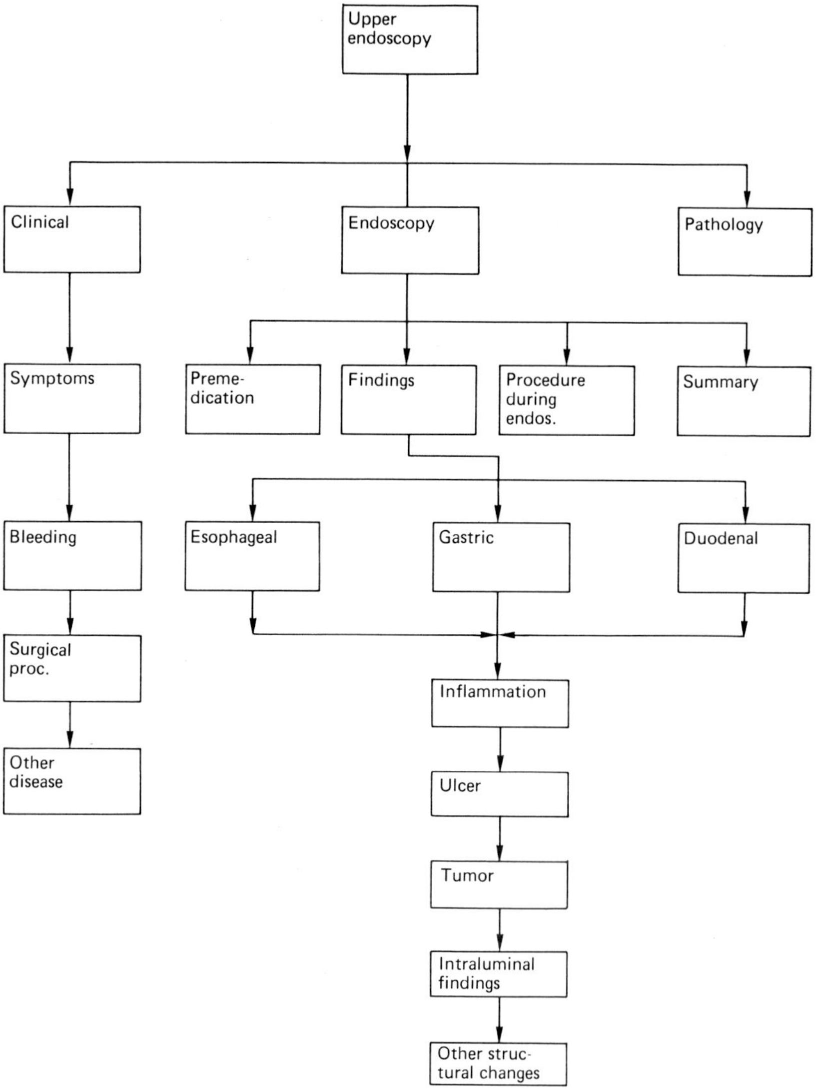

Fig. 3. Flow chart of endoscopy procedures.

```
                                                    UPPER GI. ENDO. (2.2)(R)

      *** G. I.   B L E E D I N G ***

PAST       HISTORY OF: _  (1 = HEMATEMESIS, 2 = MELENA ONLY)
----
           NUMER OF TIMES: _
                                   YEARS    OR    MONTHS    OR    DAYS
           FIRST TIME BEFORE:       _ _            _ _             _ _

           LAST TIME BEFORE:        _ _            _ _             _ _

PRESENT    HISTORY OF: _  (1 = HEMATEMESIS, 2 = MELENA ONLY)
-------
           STARTED _ _  HOURS AGO,    STOPPED _ _  HOURS AGO

           LOWEST HB.   _ _ G,%       PRESENT HB.  _ _ G,%
--------------------------------------------------------------------------------

CHRONIC ANEMIA FOR _ _  MONTHS

USING ULCEROGENIC DRUGS  :  ASPIRIN ?  _     OTHER ANTIRHEUMATIC?  _
                            STEROIDS?  _     ALCOHOL?   _

NAMES AND DURATION OF : 1 - _ _ _ _ _ _ _ _,   _ _ _ WKS.
THE SPECIFIED DRUGS     2 - _ _ _ _ _ _ _ _,   _ _ _ WKS.  3 - _ _ _ _ _ _ _ _, _ _ _ WKS.

                                                         E. L. COMPUTERS LTD.
```

Fig. 4. One of the clinical information screens for upper GI endoscopy. The relevant possitive information is entered by inserting 'Y' (Yes) or a number.

```
                                                         UPPER GI. ENDO. (3)(R)
          ** P R E M E D I C A T I O N  &  I N S T R U M E N T S  **


PHARYNGEAL ANESTHESIA:    GARGLE? _     SPRAY? _     LOZENGE? _
        |
DRUGS:  |          SCOPOLAMINE                                              OTHER:
        | ATROPINE BUTYLBROMIDE GLUCAGON DIAZEPAM FENTANYL MEPERIDINE  _ _ _ _ _ _ _ _
--------+---------|------------|---------|---------|---------|----------|----------------
        |         |            |         |         |         |          |
MG.     | ------  |   ------   | ------  | ------  | ------  | ------   |   ------
IV./IM  |   --    |     --     |   --    |   --    |   --    |   --     |     --
        |         |            |         |         |         |          |

INSTRUMENT: _ (1 OLYMPUS    2 FUJINON    3 ACMI    4 PENTAX    5 OTHER)

  MANUFACTURER'S CODE:    FIRST INSTRUMENT: _ _ _ _ _ _    LAST INSTRUMENT: _ _ _ _ _ _

  INTUBATION:    NORMAL? _    DIFFICULT? _

                                                              E. L. COMPUTERS LTD.
```

Fig. 5. Upper GI endoscopy screen summarizing the patient preparation and choice of endoscope.

```
                                                              UPPER GI. ENDO. (11)(R)

                    ***  G A S T R I C  FINDINGS & MENU  ***

                                                                                ADD.
                  X-RAY                     ENDOSCOPY                           DETAILS
                  -----                     ---------                           -------

1. INFLAMMATION     _    NON-SPECIFIC? _    EROSIVE?        _                     _
                         ATROPHIC?     _    HYPERTROPHIC?   _                     _

2. ULCER :          _    MALIGNANT?  ___    BENIGN?   ___   UNKNOWN? ___          _

3. TUMOR :          _    MALIGNANT?  ___    BENIGN?   ___   UNKNOWN? ___          _

4. INTRALUMINAL     _    BLOOD?    _     BILE?     _      STASIS? _     FOOD? _
   FINDINGS :            VARICES?  _     BEZOAR?  ___      FOREIGN BODY? ___      _

5. POST             _    BIL. 1? _   BIL. 2? _    NEAR TOTAL GASTRECTOMY? _
   OPERATIVE :           GASTROENTEROSTOMY? _     PYLOROPLASTY?           _       _

6. STRUCTURAL       _    PROTRUSION? ___    DIVERTICULUM? ___   DILATATION? ___
   CHANGES :             NARROWING?  ___                        INELASTIC?  ___   _

                                                                  E. L. COMPUTERS LTD.
```

Fig. 6. Menu for gastric findings, by radiology and endoscopy. The findings are registered and if needed, detailed screens requested by inserting 'Y' where appropriate.

```
                                                                  UPPER GI. (11.2)(R)

                  ULCER  ==>          MALIGNANT              BENIGN           UNKNOWN
-----------------------
              |                   |
X-RAY         | REPORT            |      _                      _                 _
              | INTERPRETATION    |      _                      _                 _
-----------------------------------------------------------------------------------------
E      ==================>>
   SITE       | FUNDUS            _   UPPER 3RD BODY    _    MID 3RD BODY   _
N             | LOWER 3RD BODY    _   ANTRUM            _    PYLORUS        _
              | GREATER CURVATURE _   LESSER CURVATURE  _    ANTERIOR WALL  _
D             | POSTERIOR WALL    _   WHOLE STOMACH     _    ANASTOMOSIS    _
   -----------|--------------------------------------------------------------------------
O             | DIAM. (MM.)       __
   SIZE       | SMALL             _
S             | MEDIUM            _
              | LARGE             _
C  -AMOUNT----| SINGLE            _
              | NO.               _
O  -----------| MULTIPLE          _
   -DEPTH-----| DEPTH (MM.)       __
P             | SUPERFICIAL       _
              | MODERATE          _
Y             | DEEP              _
--------------|

                                                                  E. L. COMPUTERS LTD.
```

Fig. 7. Detailed screen for describing a gastric ulcer. The radiology report and interpretation are recorded and then the endoscopy findings. The cursor automatically goes from question to question which is answered by inserting 'Y' or a number.

UPPER GI. ENDO. (14)(R)

*** S U M M A R Y ***

EXAMINATION : DURATION _ _ MINUTES

SATISFACTORY? _ IF NOT, BECAUSE OF: POOR COOPERATION? _ STASIS? _
INCOMPLETE EXAM.? _ EQUIPMENT FAILURE? _
UNCLEAR FINDINGS? _

COMPLICATIONS? _ : ALLERGIC? _ CARDIOVASCULAR? _ ASPIRATION? _
PERFORATION? _ BLEEDING? _ DEATH? _ OTHER? _ _ _ _ _ _ _ _ _

FOR G. I. BLEEDING - SOURCE:_ _ _ _ _ _ _ _ _ _ _ _ _ _ _ _ _ _ _

ADDITIONAL REMARKS: _

EXAMINATION PERFORMED BY: TRAINEE? _ SPECIALIST? _
NAMES: DR. _ _ _ _ _ _ _ _ _, _ _ _ _ _ _ _ _ _

IF EXAM COMPLETED, ENTER DATE: DAY _ _ MONTH _ _ YEAR _ _

E. L. COMPUTERS LTD.

Fig. 8. Summary of endoscopic examination, complications and examiners. Filling in the date closes the file, additions can be made but not changes.

COLON SCREENING FILE(R)

ID :

*** (B) F A M I L Y H I S T O R Y ***

	FIRST DEGREE RELATIVES				SECOND DEGREE RELATIVES					
					MATERNAL			PATERNAL		
	F	M	CHILDREN	SIBS	GM	GF	UNCLE AUNT	GM	GF	UNCLE AUNT
(1) COLON TUMORS	1	2	3	4	5	6	7	8	9	10
1. COLON CANCER	_	_	_	_	_	_	_	_	_	_
2. BENIGN COLON POLYP	_	_	_	_	_	_	_	_	_	_
3. FAMILIAL POLYPOSIS	_	_	_	_	_	_	_	_	_	_
4. JUVENILE POLYP	_	_	_	_	_	_	_	_	_	_
(2) NON-COLON GI TUMORS										
1. MOUTH,PHARYNX,ESOPH.	_	_	_	_	_	_	_	_	_	_
2. STOMACH	_	_	_	_	_	_	_	_	_	_
3. SMALL BOWEL	_	_	_	_	_	_	_	_	_	_
4. PANCREATIC, BILIARY	_	_	_	_	_	_	_	_	_	_
5. HEPATIC (+METASTATIC)	_	_	_	_	_	_	_	_	_	_

E. L. COMPUTERS LTD.

Fig. 9. One of the detailed screens from the Colon Tumor Screening Program for describing the family history of cancer. Data entry can be direct into the computer or by using the code numbers for batch processing.

```
                                                        COLON SCREENING FILE(R)
ID :

        *** (2) S I G M O I D O S C O P Y ***

(1) EXAMINER : DR. _ _ _ _ _ _ _ _ _ _ _ _ _ _ _    DATE:  DAY _ _   MONTH _ _   YEAR _ _

(2) INSTRUMENT: 1. OLYMPUS CF-1TS? _        2. OLYMPUS CF-MB? _
                2. OLYMPUS TCF-IS? _        3. RIGID? _    5. OTHER? _ _ _ _ _ _ _ _ _ _ _

(3) DISTANCE EXAMINED _ _ CM.

(4) FINDINGS:   1. NORMAL? _  2. HEMORRHOIDS? _   3. POLYP < 0.5 CM? _
                4. POLYP  > 0.5 CM? __  5. MULTIPLE POLYPS  > 0.5 CM? _
                6. CANCER? _    7. INADEQUATE EXAM.? _   8. ULCERATIVE COLITIS? _
                9. CROHN'S DISEASE? _     10. IBD, TYPE UNCERTAIN? _   11. _ _ _ _ _ _ _ _

(5) SITE:       1. RECTUM? _   2. SIGMOID? _   3. DESCENDING COLON? _

(6) PATHOLOGY NO. _ _ _ _ - _ _
          1. HYPERPLASTIC POLYP? _     2. TUBULAR ADENOMA? _    3. VILLOUS ADENOMA? _
          4. MIXED ADENOMA? _    5. CANCER? _   6. ULCERATIVE COLITIS? _
          7. CROHN'S DISEASE? _    8. IBD, TYPE UNCERTAIN? _    9. _ _ _ _ _ _ _ _ _ _ _ _

                                                           E. L. COMPUTERS LTD.
```

Fig. 10. Screen from the Colon Tumor Screening Program for entering the results of the sigmoidoscopic examination. Data entry can be direct or via the code numbers.

Data entry of other endoscopic procedures, e.g. lower endoscopy, is similar to the above. However, this on-line data entry system is not practical for a preventive medicine project, such as colon cancer screening. This project is based on medical interviewing, diagnostic procedures, pathology reports and even the results of surgery in selected cases. The results are integrated into a structured, coded worksheet based on prepared options. This data-entry form is then rapidly transferred to the computer by entering the data code; the accuracy of data entry is easily confirmed by visualizing screens based word-for-word on the data-entry forms (fig. 9, 10). Again, a printed summary is immediately available for the referring physician.

Programs Available and Costs

Most of the programs listed in table II, A, B and E are available or being developed. Changes and improvements are constantly being made as experience accumulates and innovations occur in the practice of gastroenterology. The minicomputer hardware and programs will probably cost $20,000 to $40,000 depending on the configuration chosen and sharing of costs. For users requiring only summarized data management, a microcomputer and abbreviated software is adequate. The costs would then range between $5,000 and $10,000.

Future Developments

The introduction of computer technology into clinical gastroenterology must be gradual and in defined areas in order to gain experience and overcome the negative attitude of the more established physicians to working directly with a computer terminal. We must be careful not to disappoint by being overambitious! Once data management of the endoscopy services is accepted the other fields open to exploration include: diagnosis, investigation and treatment decision analysis; and management of GI clinics. Both of these topics are dealt with in other chapters of this book. It is important, in the area of decision analysis, that computer technology be looked upon as a means of guidance to the physician and not as a potential competitor. Many of the programs, as described by *de Dombal* (pp. 119–133) [8], can be based on the data bank derived from the experience of each GI department and are quite easily managed by a minicomputer. However, the vast amount of data generated by an active GI clinic, if not handled selectively, can easily overwhelm the computer system by its mere volume, both in the time needed for data entry and by the large disk area taken for storage. In this case, integration of the minicomputer into a larger system may be necessary.

References

1 Döbrönte, Z.; Náfrádi, J.; Varró, V.; Benedek, S.: Computer aided data processing for digestive endoscopy with the help of a code-system. Endoscopy *7*: 1–5 (1975).

2 Frühmorgen, P.: Documentation of endoscopic findings; in Frühmorgen, Classen, Endoscopy and biopsy in gastroenterology: technique and indications, pp. 24–34 (Springer, New York 1980).

3 Gorry, G.A.: The personal computer and clinical practise (Editorial). Archs intern. Med. *141*: 1745–1746 (1981).

4 Kanzler, G. von; Giere, W.; Arndt, F.J.: Programmierte Befundschreibung – Rationelle Dokumentation und Auswertung proktologischer Untersuchungen über EDV. Z. Gastroenterol. *10*: 567–574 (1972).

5 Macrae, F.A.; Williams, C.B.: A prospective colonoscopic follow-up study of 500 adenoma patients with multivariate analysis to predict risk of subsequent colorectal tumors (Abstract). Gastroenterology *82*: 1122 (1982).
6 Pancotto, F.S.; Manning, A.P.; Garbutt, J.T., Jr.: Computer generated endoscopy reports: a method for developing a data bank of digestive diseases (Abstract). Gastrointest. Endosc. *27*: 127 (1981).
7 Pauker, S.G.; Kassirer, J.P.: Clinical decision analysis by personal computer. Archs intern. Med. *141*: 1831–1837 (1981).
8 Rozen, P.: Computer assistance in gastroenterology: a review. Clin. Gastroenterol. *4*: 403–414 (1982).
9 Rozen, P.; Fireman, Z.; Terdiman, R.; Hellerstein, S.J.; Rattan, J.; Gilat, T.: Selective screening for colorectal tumors in the Tel-Aviv area: Technique and initial results; in Winawer, Schottenfeld, Sherlock, Colorectal cancer: prevention, epidemiology and screening, pp. 285–298 (Raven Press, New York 1980).
10 Rozen, P.; Gilat, T.; Levy, E.: Computer assistance for gastrointestinal endoscopy units. Gastrointest. Endosc. *28*: 111–112 (1982).
11 Stalnikowicz, R.: Computer aided data processing for upper digestive endoscopy with the help of a code system; doctorate thesis supervised by P. Rozen, Tel-Aviv (1977).
12 Series/I Digest; 5th ed. (IBM Corporation, Technical Publications Department, Atlanta 1981).
13 Ward, M.: Microcomputer data storage and analysis for clinical audit. Aust. clin. Rev. *3*: 16–21 (1981).

P. Rozen, MD, Gastroenterology Department, Ichilov Hospital, 6 Weizman Street, Tel Aviv 64239 (Israel)

Front. gastrointest. Res., vol. 7, pp. 110–118 (Karger, Basel 1984)

Interviewing by Paramedics with Computer Analysis: Gastrointestinal Cancer

Susan E. Clamp, Janet S. Wenham

Clinical Information Science Group, St. James Hospital, Leeds, England

Introduction

Gastrointestinal cancer is a common complaint in most developed countries, responsible (in the UK alone) for around 20,000 deaths per annum. Survival (on the whole rather poor) appears to depend upon the *extent of disease at treatment*. Unfortunately, however, there is considerable evidence of delay between onset of symptoms, presentation to the doctor, and diagnosis – ranging up to a median value of 46 weeks in some instances [5].

In theory therefore some kind of 'screening' or 'case-finding' procedure would thus seem desirable, and since identification of asymptomatic disease (via serological markers and similar techniques) is currently in its infancy [1], case finding (i.e. earlier diagnosis of symptomatic disease) would seem to offer the only immediate practical means of reducing mortality.

Several techniques are available – ranging from wide employment of endoscopic examination, through detailed clinical interview and examination to simple feacal occult blood testing. Currently available evidence, however, suggests that an *integrated* approach is optimal, with a large (albeit selected) population receiving some kind of simple "screening procedure' – this procedure then being used to select patients at "high risk' for subsequent intensive (high-technology) investigation.

Of course this concept in turn poses problems. If clinical interview is to be included as part of the 'first screen', then the interview has to be carried out in such a way as to obtain a reliable and reproducible version of each patient's symptoms. The problem is that in the foreseeable future many countries will almost certainly not be able to mobilise the resources for such interviews to be carried out by medically qualified persons. Accordingly, over the last 10 years we have been undertaking a series of experiments to determine (a) whether *paramedical* personnel can interview patients with gastrointestinal symptoms, and (b) when this interview is subjected to subsequent analysis by computer if the resultant analysis is useful. In this chapter, we set out our experience, and comment on some of the wider implications.

Physicians Assistants and Paramedics

Until the early 1960s, the idea that persons other than physicians could interview patients (and obtain sensible clinical data from them) was frowned upon by the medical profession as a whole. However, about 20 years ago – partly as a result of the availability of ex-armed-services paramedical personnel, and partly as a result of the increasing work load for frontline clinicians – a number of workers began to study the possibility of safely and effectively delegating some of these (hitherto sacrosanct) functions to non-physicians.

Chief amongst these early pioneers was Dr. *Eugene Stead* of Duke University, N.C.; some idea of the rapid progress of this concept can be gained by recalling that in 1965 4 candidates presented for the Duke University Physicians Assistant Course, whereas by 1971 over 1,000 candidates were attending courses in Washington and Maryland alone.

There has thus been a rapid acceptance of the concept of the 'physician's assistant', a person to whom some of the functions of data gathering can be safely delegated. Two types of physicians assistant have emerged. The first is trained broadly (but perhaps superficially) to obtain histories from patients with virtually any medical complaint, and is also trained to make some simple medical decisions. Such persons are increasingly useful in remote areas.

The second type (with which we deal here), is a paramedical person trained *in-depth* in one specific area (in this case gastroenterological symptomatology) and trained for a specific purpose (namely data gathering), with clinical decision-making being left entirely in the hands of the medical profession. Such an approach, in our experience, is more acceptable to doctors in general, and could be seen to offer some advantage – in that, in terms of rapidity of training and decreased cost of employment, this type of person consumes far less resources per patient screened than does a qualified doctor.

Computer Specifications and Use

Specifications for the type of computer to be used in such studies stem directly from the nature of the screening procedure. By definition: (1) the screening procedure needs to be widespread, and therefore multiple computers (or terminals) are necessary. (2) The screening should be as cost-effective as can be achieved, and hence the computer should be as small as possible and particularly as cheap as possible. (3) The computer will be used mainly by inexperienced personnel, and therefore the system must be reliable and easy to use – so that training in terms of computer usage can be kept to a minimum.

In practical terms this implies that a modern microcomputer (such as a Pet 8032 or Apple II or their successors) is perfectly adequate for this sort of usage. It is therefore preferable to mainframe or minicomputers on the grounds of cost, availability, reliability and particularly ease of usage by inexperienced computer users.

Specific Mode of Use

In the studies to be described (and most allied studies) the computer has been used in the fashion described elsewhere in this book [*de Dombal*, p. 119]. First a clinically qualified doctor identifies a suitable candidate for 'screening'. A case history is then obtained by a paramedical person from the patient with gastrointestinal symptoms, using the structured data collection sheet in figure 1. These data are then coded and entered into the microcomputer, so that they may be compared with the symptoms of several hundred other patients via a Bayesian analysis – the resultant printout (fig. 2) being visible within 2–3min. As regards hardware, a variety of computers have been used in our own studies (Wang 2200T, Pet 8032, Apple II) – but since the simple Bayesian program is written in elementary BASIC and accommodates less than 16KB it is virtually machine-independent.

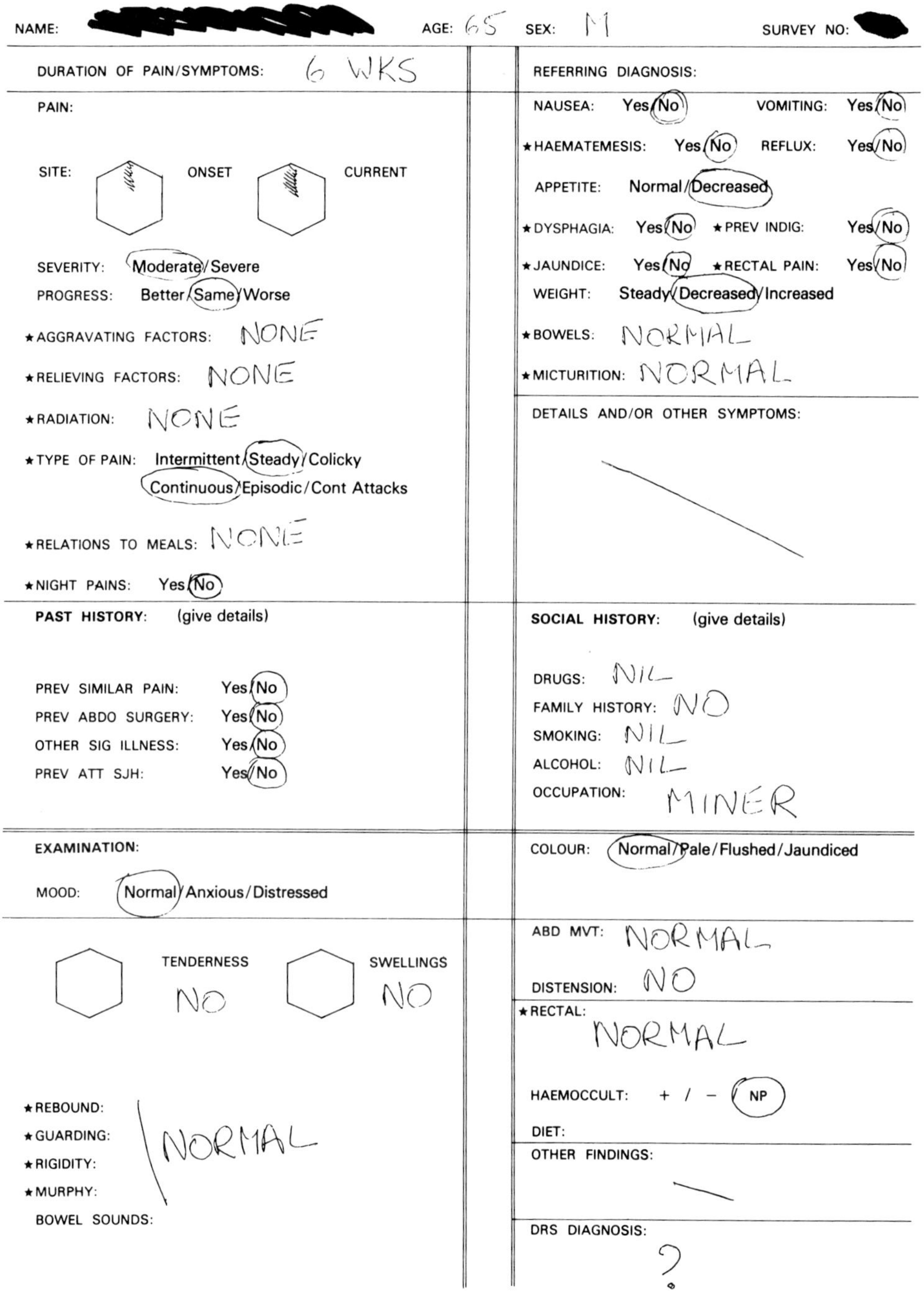

NAME: [redacted] AGE: 65 SEX: M SURVEY NO: [redacted]

DURATION OF PAIN/SYMPTOMS: 6 WKS

REFERRING DIAGNOSIS:

PAIN:

SITE: ONSET CURRENT

SEVERITY: Moderate/Severe

PROGRESS: Better/Same/Worse

★AGGRAVATING FACTORS: NONE

★RELIEVING FACTORS: NONE

★RADIATION: NONE

★TYPE OF PAIN: Intermittent/Steady/Colicky
Continuous/Episodic/Cont Attacks

★RELATIONS TO MEALS: NONE

★NIGHT PAINS: Yes/No

NAUSEA: Yes/No VOMITING: Yes/No

★HAEMATEMESIS: Yes/No REFLUX: Yes/No

APPETITE: Normal/Decreased

★DYSPHAGIA: Yes/No ★PREV INDIG: Yes/No

★JAUNDICE: Yes/No ★RECTAL PAIN: Yes/No

WEIGHT: Steady/Decreased/Increased

★BOWELS: NORMAL

★MICTURITION: NORMAL

DETAILS AND/OR OTHER SYMPTOMS:

PAST HISTORY: (give details)

PREV SIMILAR PAIN: Yes/No

PREV ABDO SURGERY: Yes/No

OTHER SIG ILLNESS: Yes/No

PREV ATT SJH: Yes/No

SOCIAL HISTORY: (give details)

DRUGS: NIL

FAMILY HISTORY: NO

SMOKING: NIL

ALCOHOL: NIL

OCCUPATION: MINER

EXAMINATION:

MOOD: Normal/Anxious/Distressed

TENDERNESS NO

SWELLINGS NO

★REBOUND:
★GUARDING:
★RIGIDITY:
★MURPHY:
BOWEL SOUNDS:
NORMAL

COLOUR: Normal/Pale/Flushed/Jaundiced

ABD MVT: NORMAL

DISTENSION: NO

★RECTAL:
NORMAL

HAEMOCCULT: + / – NP

DIET:

OTHER FINDINGS:

DRS DIAGNOSIS:
?

Fig. 1. Structured data-collection sheet utilised in Leeds studies, filled in by non-medically qualified (paramedical) personnel for susequent computer analysis.

```
CASE REF

MALE
AGE60-69
PAIN AT ONSET UPPER HALF
PAIN NOW UPPER HALF
NO RADIATION
CONTINUOUS
MODERATE
NO CHANGE
NO AGGRAV FACTORS
PAIN NOT RELATED TO FOOD
NO RELIEVING FACTORS
NO NIGHT PAINS
NO NAUSEA
NO VOMITING
NO HAEMATEMESIS
ANOREXIA
NO DYSPHAGIA
NO PREV INDIGESTION
NO JAUNDICE
NORMAL BOWELS
NORMAL MICTURITION
DECREASED WEIGHT
NO PREV SURGERY
NOT TAKING DRUGS
NO REFLUX
NO RESTROSTERNAL PAIN

OLD DATABASE
FUNCT    CHOLE    D.U.     G.U.     CANCER
  3        1       3        4        90

NEW DATABASE

FUNCT    D.U.     G.U.     CHOLE    HIATUS   CANCER
  4       0        7        2        0        86
```

Fig. 2. Computer analysis of interview data in figure 1. Such a patient would be rapidly referred for high technology investigation.

Application and Results

Hospital Studies

During the 1970s a number of studies were carried out in hospitals, first in Leeds and subsequently elsewhere in the UK. In the initial Leeds studies [3] several hundred patients presenting to hospital with 'dyspepsia' were interviewed by a non-medically qualified physician's assistant (a computer programmer who had undergone several weeks specific training).

In these initial studies, the overall clinician's diagnostic accuracy proved to be just over 54%. Where provided with medically obtained structured data, the computer's accuracy in the same patients was 87%; and where provided with structured data obtained by the non-medically qualified physicians assistant the computer's accuracy was 81%. Where structured data obtained by physician's assistant were provided to four further doctors, their accuracy of diagnosis (in the same cases) was 74–79%.

Interestingly, the sensitivity of physicians in this series for gastric cancer was 40%, but the sensitivity of the computer, using data obtained by the physicians assistant, was 83%. Subsequent studies in Leeds showed similar results when the problem of lower gastrointestinal cancer was studied. Physician's sensitivity for colorectal cancer [2] proved to be somewhat higher (74.7% on clinical data alone and 93% after investigations). Nevertheless, the computer sensitivity (90.9% on clinical data alone) appeared to offer some potential advantage in terms of case finding and screening studies.

During the latter part of the 1970s further groups in the UK conducted similar studies with confirmatory results. In particular studies at Airedale District General Hospital, 30 miles west of Leeds [4] and at Bristol in the South West of England [7] showed comparable sensitivity for gastro-intestinal cancer. Similar studies carried out in Glasgow, Scotland, showed equally encouraging results; and the recent World Congress of Gastro-Enterology heard from *Li Zeng-lie and Hu Fu-lie* [6] that comparable studies have been carried out in China with results (in over 1,000 patients) closely parallelling the UK results already outlined.

It would appear therefore that, once in hospital, cases of gastro-intestinal cancer can be identified (relatively effectively) by computer analysis of data obtained by non-medically qualified persons. However, it will also be rapidly apparent that such a service would fail to solve the problem of diagnostic delay since the majority of this occurs *before* the patient arrives at hospital.

Accordingly, in the last 3–4 years a further experiment has taken place in Leeds involving five primary health care centres and 26 general practitioners. In this study, 468 patients between the ages of 40 and 70 with gastro-intestinal symptoms (currently being seen and treated by their general practitioner) were interviewed by one of the present authors (J.S.W.). The resultant data were analysed by computer. Additionally a consultant surgeon analysed the clinical data, and faecal occult tests were performed. If *any* of these modes gave rise to concern, high technology investigations (barium studies or endoscopy) were arranged as appropriate.

Amongst the 468 patients some 23 (5%) were found to have cancer, and a further 6 to have 'malignant' colonic polyps. Table I shows the sen-

Table I. Analysis by diagnostic mode

	Cancer		*Non-cancer*	
Mode	true positive	false negative	false positive	true negative
All	26	1	195	219
Clinician	17	10	125	298
Nurse + computer	22	5	74	340
Nurse + FOB + computer	23	4	83	331

Results of diagnostic 'screening' study in Leeds in 468 patients seen in five primary health care centres (27 of whom were subsequently found to have cancer of the gastro-intestinal tract.)

sitivity of each diagnostic mode for cancer, as well as the specificity. It will be seen that *overall* this mode of analysis was highly effective in detecting gastro-intestinal cancer – though at the expense of a high false-positive rate. Table I also shows that the *computer analysis of data obtained by a nursing sister was highly effective* – identifying more cancers than the physician alone, and at the cost of 50 fewer false-positive investigations.

From these studies it is possible to conclude that – although whole population screening for gastro-intestinal cancer might be impractical – case finding (by means of a non-medically qualified person's interview analysed by computer and coupled with faecal occult blood tests) might well have a part to play in reducing the delay in diagnosing this common disease.

Cost Effectiveness

Before such a conclusion can be asserted, however, several questions need to be raised concerning cost-effectiveness of the type of procedure outlined. These may be summarised as follows:

(1) Is the Procedure Effective? The evidence outlined above, coupled with the evidence from Airedale, Bristol, and China, would seem to indicate that computer analysis of a non-physician-obtained case history (taken in a structured format) is reasonably effective in detecting gastro-intestinal

cancer at an early stage. It appears that 80% of gastro-intestinal cancers can be so detected, with a false-positive rate of about 20%. These figures are considerably more effective than the current performance of the unaided clinician. This procedure will not detect (by definition) asymptomatic disease; but in the Leeds studies the delay between presentation and diagnosis was reduced from a median of approximately 6 months to a median of 31 days.

(2) Effect on Survival? When the effect on survival is considered, the picture which emerges is less encouraging. In particular, in the Leeds studies, there was no effect upon survival of upper gastro-intestinal cancer whatsoever. It can be argued that early detection of symptomatic disease improves the quality of life for these patients; but in terms of survival it would appear that the only method likely to be effective in prolonging life is detection of cancer before symptomatic presentation to the doctor.

In the lower gastro-intestinal tract, the position is more encouraging. The detection in our series of several early colorectal cancers coupled with the finding of six (malignant) polyps gives rise to some grounds for optimism. However, even here it will be several years before any firm conclusions can be drawn. Nevertheless, the evidence is already sufficient to enter a suitable caveat. If the objective is cancer detection, then the procedures outlined above are effective. If the objective is prolongation of life, then the procedures outlined above may not be effective.

(3) Cost? Surprisingly, it turns out that the procedures outlined above, although far cheaper than the conventional clinical interview, are still quite costly. The chief element of cost in this system is the salary of the nursing sister, and – on a wide scale – effectiveness is limited by the relatively small number of patients (about ten) which can be interviewed in any one session by a single paramedical person without becoming bored or fatigued. Accordingly, further studies are underway in Leeds using simple patient questionnaires in an attempt to achieve the type of results outlined in the above paragraphs by (1) computer analysis of patient-completed structured questionnaires coupled with (2) faecal occult blood testing.

We would contend that if the results of these current studies show little or no degradation of accuracy (in terms of sensitivity and specificity for cancer) then the procedures we have described would be a highly effective, and cost-efficient, means of improving the service offered to the patients with gastro-intestinal cancer.

References

1 Cotton, P.B.: Early gastric cancer. Proc. 2nd BSG Int. Workshop, 1981.
2 Dombal, F.T. de; Clamp, S.E.; Leaper, D.J.; Staniland, J.R.; Horrocks, C.: Computer-aided diagnosis of lower gastro-intestinal tract disorders. Gastroenterology *68*: 252–260 (1975).
3 Horrocks, J.C.; Dombal, F.T. de: Diagnosis of dyspepsia using data collected by a non-medically qualified physicians assistant. Br. med. J. *iii*: 421–423 (1975).
4 Horrocks, J.C.; Lambert, D.E.; McAdam, W.A.F.; Morgan, A.G.; Pacsoo, C.; Darnborough, A.; Dombal, F.T. de: Transfer of computer-aided diagnosis of dyspepsia from one geographical area to another. Gut *17*: 640–644 (1976).
5 MacAdam, D.B.: A study in general practice of the symptoms and delay patterns in the diagnosis of gastrointestinal cancer. J. R. Coll. gen. Pract. *29*: 723–729 (1979).
6 Zeng-lie, L.; Fu-le, H.: Computer-aided diagnosis of gastric cancer. Chinese med. J. *65*: 293–296 (1982).
7 Zoltie, N.; Horrocks, J.C.; Dombal, F.T. de: Computer-aided diagnosis of dyspepsia – reports on transferability of a system with emphasis on early diagnosis of gastric cancer. Meth. Inf. Med. *16*: 89–92 (1977).

S.E. Clamp, BA, O.U., Research Assistant, Clinical Information Science Group, Department of Surgery, St. James Hospital, Leeds LS9 7TF (England)

Front. gastrointest. Res., vol. 7, pp. 119–133 (Karger, Basel 1984)

Computers and Decision-Making: An Overview for Gastro-Enterologists

F.T. de Dombal

Clinical Information Science Group, The University of Leeds, Leeds, England

Introduction

The application of computers to decision-making in clinical practice has been frequently described as being amongst the most controversial in the whole of computer usage. Indeed, this topic has attracted more polemic and partly informed comment than all other medical applications of computers combined. On the one hand, it is argued that 'human life is too important to be trusted to the computer' – a manifestly fallacious argument for anyone to make who has entrusted his or her own life to a scheduled airline flight. On the other hand, it is argued (frequently and with some force!) that doctors are manifestly inefficient, their practice is rooted in mystique rather than science, and in some 'Luddite' fashion they are unwilling to accept the challenge of technology – once again a manifestly fallacious argument when we consider the ubiquitous high technology of modern medicine.

It will be apparent nevertheless that the application of computers to decision-making in gastro-enterology raises a number of fundamental problems; and it may therefore be as well to deal with these problems before describing individual systems and individual instances of application.

Fundamental Problems

Diagnostic Aid or Surrogate Diagnostician?

Perhaps the most important problem concerns the basic role of the computer in the diagnostic process. Is the computer to be the diagnostic *agent*? Or should the computer act merely as a diagnostic *aid* – analysing symptoms in the same way as a blood test analyses red cells, or an ECG analyses electrical activity – and one which can be over-ridden by the doctor?

Increasingly in the last 20 years opinion has swung in favour of the latter of these modes. In the early 1960s systems designed to *replace* the doctor as a decision-maker were constructed; and have almost universally been rejected. Partly this was due to the primitive technology of the time but mostly this was due to the point-blank refusal of doctors to accept machines which suborned their traditional role.

Indeed, there is cogent argument to support this latter viewpoint on the part of the medical profession. It can be claimed with some justification that many of the attributes of patients which a doctor routinely elicits 'by osmosis' (such as the 'look' or 'feel' of the patient) cannot currently be quantified and entered into any existing computer system. Moreover, it can be argued with equal justification that only a human being (in this case a doctor) is capable of taking a 'wholistic' view of the situation and assess such imponderable aspects in decision-making as the value or 'utility' of a treatment to a particular patient. For these reasons (as *Lusted* [4] and others have pointed out for many years), talk of 'computer decisions' or 'computer doing diagnosis' is not helpful. What is feasible at this time is computer *assistance* for doctors making decisions about patients; in this adjunctive role there has recently been some modest advance, and (apparently) useful systems have begun to emerge.

Mode of Action

The next major problem which has exercised those working in the field over the last 10 years concerns the basic mode of action of the system designed to aid the doctor. Once the role is defined (as discussed above) two questions in particular have emerged in the production of computer aids for decision-making. These can be summarised as follows: (1) Knowledge engineering versus brute force? (2) Source of computer data?

The first of these questions can be summed up as follows. Should the computer produce a diagnostic or decision-making prediction by means of 'knowledge engineering?' That is to say, should *artificial intelligence* techniques be involved so that the computer will in some way 'think like a doctor'.

Proponents of this view [1–3] have usually favoured *'rule-based systems'* where a series of simple 'rules' are fed into the computer – which then attempts to analyse each new case by working through the rules in turn until a diagnostic possibility emerges. It is claimed that doctors think this way. On the other hand, the proponents of the 'brute force' approach [4, 5] claim that it is currently almost impossible to make a computer think like a doctor, and in any case it is undesirable. Their approach uses the 'brute force' of the computer to perform the function for which it is best suited (holding and analysing large amounts of data). The 'brute force' proponents contend that when this computer strength is allied to different (human) strengths, an optimal system emerges.

The second question concerns the source of data to be used by the computer in making its prediction. One school of thought has contended that what is required is a series of *'expert' or 'peer' judgements* to be held within the computer. The advantages claimed are (a) that the computer will then possess 'the best of clinical knowledge', and (b) that it is relatively easy to derive such a data base by asking experts what they think. The alternative point of view suggests that 'experts' may not always be ideally suited to this task, may have difficulty verbalising their own rules, and even more difficulty in allocating numbers and weightings to clinical attributes. Moreover, since 'expert' opinion varies, all that may be achieved by an expert system is the codification of a particular experts view. In many areas of medicine no consensus viewpoint exists – and it is argued that the computer would be better to rely on *observed findings in real patients* rather than (possibly unreliable) expert opinion.

Mathematical Models

It is not proposed in this chapter to discuss mathematical models in great detail. Other (excellent) expositions on this subject can be readily found by the interested reader [4, 6]. However, some brief outline may be helpful. The so-called 'artificial intelligence' approach has usually relied on some kind of *decision tree* (fig. 1) in which a series of pertinent questions direct the computer (and thus the human) to an appropriate diagnosis. The principal technique employed by proponents of 'brute force' is 'Bayesian' analysis: that is the use of a mathematical theorem propounded by the Reverend *Thomas Bayes* in the 18th century. An example of this is shown in table I. Detailed advantages and objections to this theorem are discussed elsewhere [5].

It will be seen that the two approaches are quite different. The 'tree' approach is dependent upon a small subset of symptoms or signs, and thereby easier to understand. The Bayesian approach depends upon mathematical analysis using a large set of data and therefore is more dif-

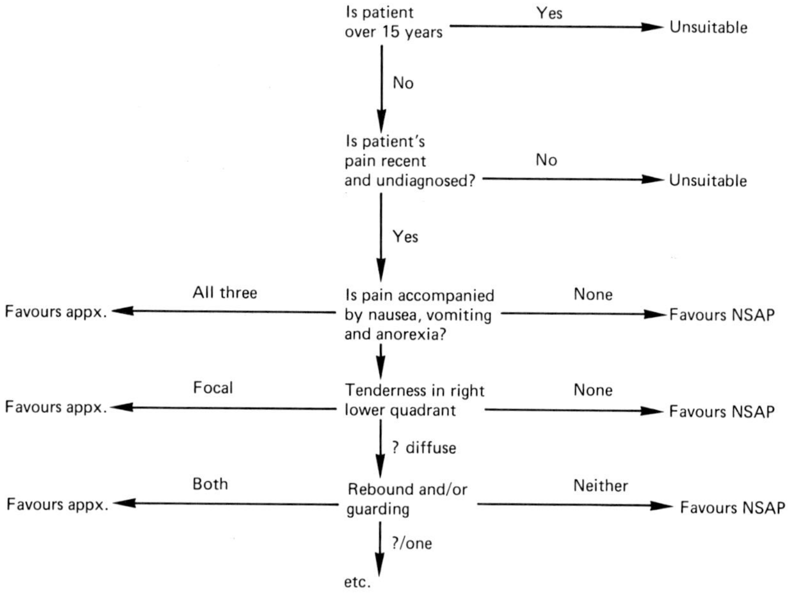

Fig. 1. Example of 'rule-based' analysis of acute abdominal pain in children. Note (a) relatively simple structure; (b) difficulty of dealing with more than two diseases or symptoms at a time, and (c) reliance upon relatively few clinical features. (Appx. = appendicitis; NSAP = nonspecific abdominal pains).

ficult to understand, particularly in terms of the numbers involved. It is, however, more 'forgiving' in that it allows at least some measure of observer variation in eliciting signs and symptoms, particularly valuable in areas of medicine where data are difficult to elicit, such as acute abdominal pain.

Hardware

The hardware employed for computer-aided decision-making in gastro-enterology has become increasingly simplified. Mainframe computers are now rarely used for this purpose, and the ubiquitous microcomputer has become established as the main vehicle for automated decision-making aid. In part, this is due to the reasons outlined above, namely that 'brute force' (such as Bayesian analysis), seems to be gaining ground as a philosophy; this approach (paradoxically) can be easily accommodated on a microcomputer. In parallel, computer developments have reduced costs dramatically and have made microcomputers vastly cheaper and easier to

Table I. Example of Bayesian analysis of acute abdominal pain in children. Note (a) large number of disease categories; (b) effect of prior probability in reducing choice; (c) how *many* features can be combined to express *balance* of probability

	Disease state						
	appx.	divert.	perf.	NSAP	chole.	SBO	panc.
(a) *'Prior' probability*[1]	24	2	2	43	9	4	2
'Conditional' probability[2]							
(b) RLQ pain	74	9	3	33	4	7	2
(c) tenderness	80	11	2	38	4	13	2
(d) Rebound tenderness	79	31	76	25	36	28	44
Total (a×b×c×d)	11,224,320	6,138	912	1,348,050	864	10,192	352
'Posterior' probability[3], %	89.1	0.1	0.1	10.7	0.1	0.1	0.1

appx. = Appendicitis; divert. = diverticulosis; perf. = perforation; chole. = cholecystitis; panc. = pancreatitis; RLQ = right lower quadrant; NSAP = nonspecific abdominal pain; SBO = small bowel obstruction.

[1] Prevalence of disease in general population (e.g. 24% of all patients have appendicitis).

[2] Prevalence of each symptom in each disease (e.g. 74% of appx. patients have RLQ pain).

[3] For each disease, total for that disease/total for all diseases (e.g. for appx. 11, 224,320/ 12,590,828).

use than hitherto. Finally, data held in microcomputers are more secure (an important point where patient data is concerned) and, as a result, most decision-making systems in use at the present time in gastro-enterology employ one or other of the currently popular microcomputers.

A Modern System

It may help in understanding computer aid to decision-making to describe briefly a single modern system, its philosophy, and its usage in a number of centres.

General Principles

Figure 2 illustrates the general principles of what needs to be done if a computer system is to be used to aid diagnosis, in this instance the diagnosis of acute abdominal pain. Data from a 'new' patient must be obtained

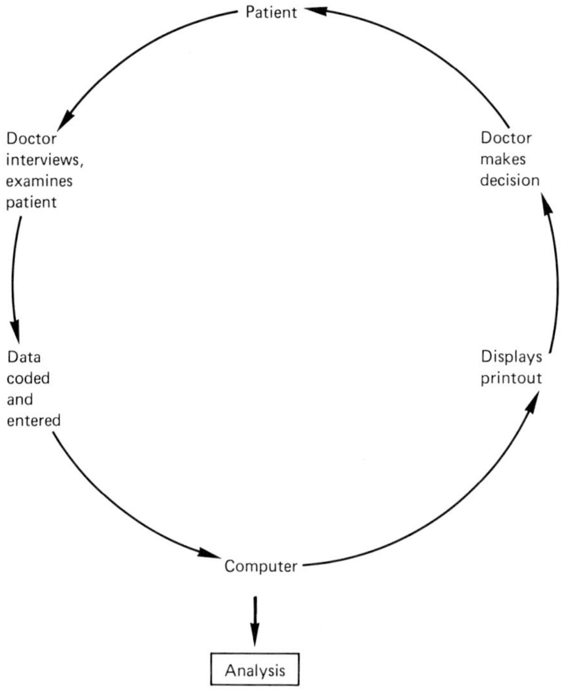

Fig. 2. General principles of computer-aided diagnosis. The computer is aiding the doctor, guiding and teaching, but in no way replacing the doctor, or the doctor's decision. From *Horrocks* [9].

from the patient by the doctor, coded, and entered into the computer. It then performs an analysis upon the data from the 'new' patient (comparing the data with those of several thousand others by means of a Bayesian analysis). The computer then displays some kind of information to the doctor, following which the clinician (and not the computer) makes a decision about therapy.

It will thus be seen that the role of the computer in this system is ancillary, and merely provides one additional 'special investigation' for the doctor to consider whilst deciding what to do about the case in question.

Data-Collection

Crucial to the whole exercise is the question of the data elicited from each patient, and many systems have foundered because the data collected were inadequate, inaccurate, unreliable or intrinsically unhelpful. The first

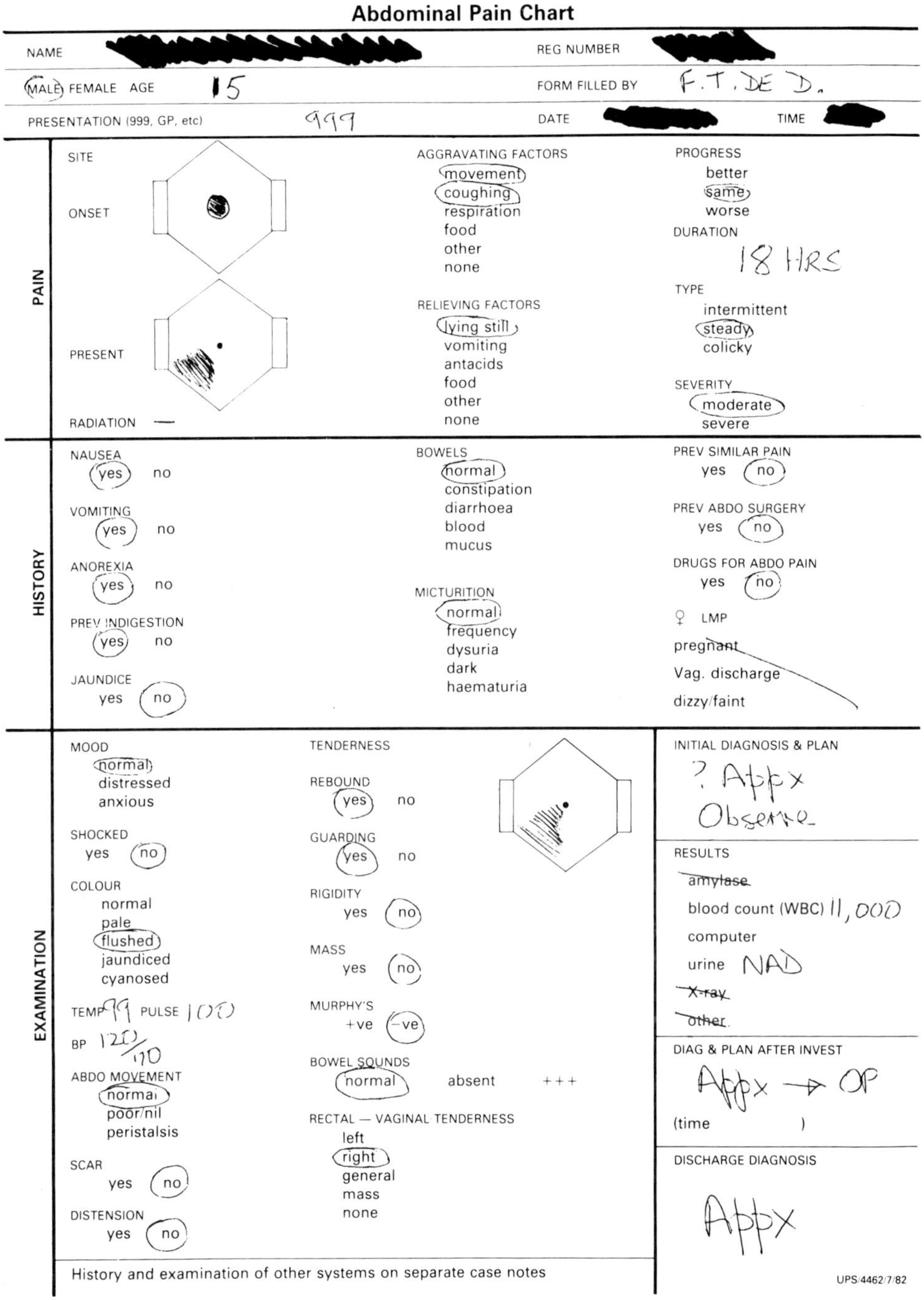

Abdominal Pain Chart

NAME [redacted] REG NUMBER [redacted]

MALE FEMALE AGE 15 FORM FILLED BY F.T. DE D.

PRESENTATION (999, GP, etc) 999 DATE [redacted] TIME [redacted]

PAIN

SITE

ONSET

PRESENT

RADIATION —

AGGRAVATING FACTORS
movement
coughing
respiration
food
other
none

RELIEVING FACTORS
lying still
vomiting
antacids
food
other
none

PROGRESS
better
same
worse

DURATION
18 HRS

TYPE
intermittent
steady
colicky

SEVERITY
moderate
severe

HISTORY

NAUSEA
yes no

VOMITING
yes no

ANOREXIA
yes no

PREV INDIGESTION
yes no

JAUNDICE
yes no

BOWELS
normal
constipation
diarrhoea
blood
mucus

MICTURITION
normal
frequency
dysuria
dark
haematuria

PREV SIMILAR PAIN
yes no

PREV ABDO SURGERY
yes no

DRUGS FOR ABDO PAIN
yes no

♀ LMP
pregnant
Vag. discharge
dizzy/faint

EXAMINATION

MOOD
normal
distressed
anxious

SHOCKED
yes no

COLOUR
normal
pale
flushed
jaundiced
cyanosed

TEMP 99 PULSE 100

BP 120/70

ABDO MOVEMENT
normal
poor/nil
peristalsis

SCAR
yes no

DISTENSION
yes no

TENDERNESS

REBOUND
yes no

GUARDING
yes no

RIGIDITY
yes no

MASS
yes no

MURPHY'S
+ve −ve

BOWEL SOUNDS
normal absent +++

RECTAL — VAGINAL TENDERNESS
left
right
general
mass
none

INITIAL DIAGNOSIS & PLAN
? Appx
Observe

RESULTS
amylase
blood count (WBC) 11,000
computer
urine NAD
X-ray
other.

DIAG & PLAN AFTER INVEST
Appx → OP
(time)

DISCHARGE DIAGNOSIS
Appx

History and examination of other systems on separate case notes

UPS/4462/7/82

Fig. 3. Example of data collection form used in the National Trial of Computer-Aided Diagnosis of Acute Abdominal Pain.

task of creating such a system is thus to define the clinical attributes to be collected and make sure that this collection can be done as reliably as possible.

Figure 3 shows an example of such a data collection form, designed to record data from a patient with acute abdominal pain. Actually the form comes in two sheets. Data is recorded by the doctor on the top form, and (via 'no carbon required' paper) a copy is automatically generated on the second form, which is then used for entering data into the computer. As shown, the second form (though not the first) has a series of code numbers, so that data can be easily entered.

Three points are worth making. First, the top form is as simple as possible and enables the doctor collecting data to record his findings in the minimum time and with maximum clarity. Second, the whole of the form, the categories involved and the definitions of these categories, result from detailed consultation with well over 100 doctors, mostly consulting sur-

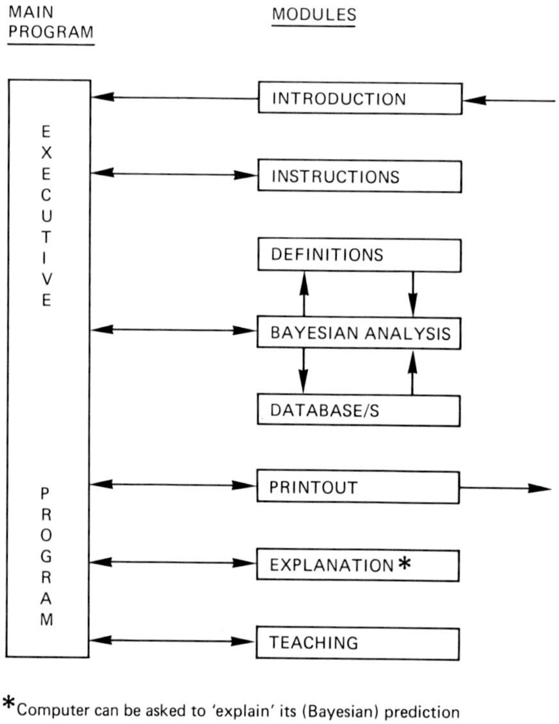

Fig. 4. Block diagram of computer diagnostic program used in the National Trial (see text).

geons in a variety of centres around the world. Third, the 'top' sheet is so designed that it becomes part of the permanent case record – a very important point since doctors are understandably reluctant to 'do things twice' – once for real and once for the computer!

Computer Analysis

Figure 4 demonstrates some points of this analysis. As will be seen, although the basic computer program follows the outline of philosophy discussed above, 'chained' to the basic program are a series of modules which: (a) introduce the system to the doctor; (b) offer the doctor guidance about the use of the system; (c) offer the doctor assistance with definitions of terms; (d) offer guidance concerning interpretation of the computer printout, and (e) offer additional teaching packages.

A sample of computer printout is illustrated in figure 5. The figure is self-explanatory, and provides a good summary of the usage of the computer in the case in question. Again (as with any other special investigation) the computer printout becomes part of the permanent case record.

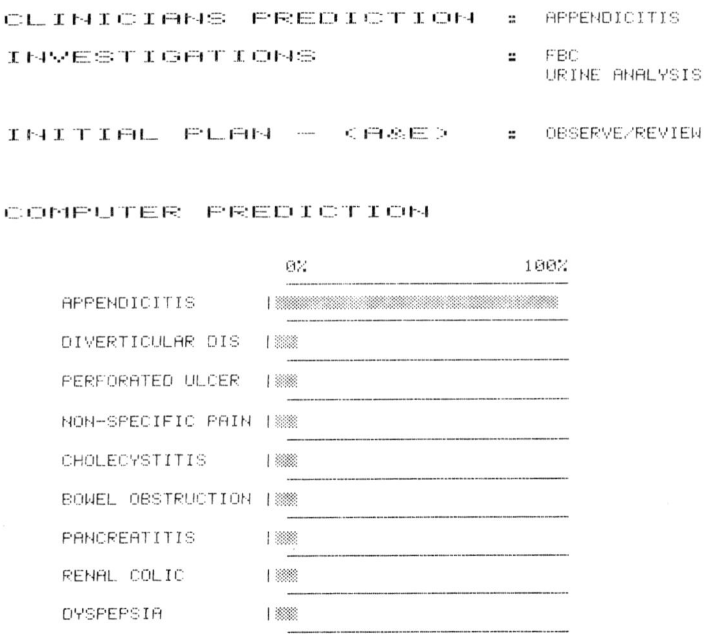

Fig. 5. Printout from microcomputer relating to data entered via data collection forms (fig. 2).

COMPUTER-AIDED DIAGNOSIS PROGRAM

ACUTE ABDOMINAL PAIN

This is an experimental programme to help you make accurate diagnoses.
CLINICAL JUDGEMENT MUST ALWAYS TAKE PRECEDENCE

COMPUTER user is : F.T. DE DOMBAL (Consultant)
DATA from : User

Patient's Reg.No : [redacted]
Date : [redacted] at [redacted] hrs.

SYMPTOMS

MALE
AGE10-19
PAIN ONSET CENTRAL
PAIN NOW RLQ
AGGRAV BY MOVT
AGGRAV BY COUGH
RELIEF-LYING
NO CHANGE
PAIN 12-24 HRS
STEADY NOW
MODERATE
NAUSEA
VOMITING
ANOREXIA
PREV INDIGESTION
NO JAUNDICE
BOWELS NORMAL
MICTURITION NORMAL
NO PREV SIMILAR PAIN
NO PREV ABD SURGERY
NOT TAKING DRUGS

EXAMINATION

NORMAL MOOD
FLUSHED
ABDO.MVT.NORMAL
NO SCARS
NO DISTENSION
TENDER RLQ
REBOUND
GUARDING
NO RIGIDITY
NO SWELLINGS
MURPHY -VE
NORMAL BOWEL SOUNDS
TENDER RT PR

Following receipt of the printout, the doctor then confirms his original diagnosis and decision (or may alter either in the light of the computer prediction – again as with any other special investigation). In practice, most hospitals using such a system have adopted a format of use whereby – if the computer agrees with the doctor – he proceeds with treatment. If the computer prediction does *not* match the doctor's own prediction, then before proceeding the doctor calls in a more senior colleague. Should the resultant consultation over-ride the computer's prediction then this is perfectly acceptable. Indeed, as stated on the printout (q.v.), clinical judgement *must* take precedence.

Use of System

One major problem with computer-aided diagnostic and decision-making systems concerns their evaluation. Such systems are difficult to evaluate, and in many cases little or no evaluation has been undertaken.

Table II. Initial findings of Leeds system [8]. Note that (a) LOW initial clinical diagnostic accuracy (normal); (b) HIGH computer accuracy (irrelevant); (c) HIGH accuracy of senior clinicians/registrars/house surgeons (crucial)

Category	% accuracy in consecutive series of 552 patients: Jan. 1971 to Aug. 1972
Admitting doctors	42
House surgeon (less than 6 months experience)	71
Registrar (1–2 years experience)	79
Senior clinican (over 5 years experience)	81
Computer-aided system	91

Table III. Changes in diagnostic accuracy and decision-making performance during computer-aided decision support studies [from ref. 7]

Aspect measured	Leeds (5,000 cases)	Airedale (1,500 cases)	Edinburgh (2,500 cases)
% diagnostic accuracy when patient first seen			
Before system introduced	45	54	55
After system introduced	63	65	77
% perforation rate for patients with acute appx.			
Before system introduced	36	27	25
After system introduced	10	13	10
% negative laparotomy rates			
Before system introduced	24	22	18
After system introduced	ca 10	16	10
% patients sent home in less than 24 h			
Before system introduced	20	16	19
After system introduced	40	25	34
Hospital bednights saved	> 1,000 p.a.	> 500 p.a.	> 500 p.a.

In the case of the system described above, initial evaluation soon indicated that the computer out-performed clinicians (table II). More importantly, later studies [7] indicated that clinicians themselves improved with the use of the computer both in terms of diagnosis and in terms of decision-making (table III). Of course it is relatively easy to effect such changes in the short-term, but more recent studies (table IV) have indicated that such changes are relatively long lasting. The computer system described therefore emerges not so much as a surrogate diagnostician but rather as a sophisticated and apparently effective post-graduate teaching aid.

Amenable Areas

Given from the above example that computer-aided decision-making is feasible, it may well be worth enquiring which areas of gastro-enterological practice might be amenable to computer-aided diagnosis in the not too distant future. Although in theory the whole of medicine is so amenable, in practice this is scarcely practical in the foreseeable future and some criteria can therefore be set out in order to decide which (limited) areas to study first:

There Must Be a Clinical Problem. If an area is well dealt with by current clinical method, then there is little point and little practical return in attempting to 'computerise' it.

Table IV. Showing how improved results (see tables II, III) can be maintained over a 9-year period (data from Airedale District General Hospital, Yorkshire)

	Time period		
	1973 (before system)	1976	1982
% admitting doctors accuracy	54	65	76
% Senior House Officer accuracy	60	70	82
% perforated appx rate	23	16	12
% negative laparotomy rate	27	13	8

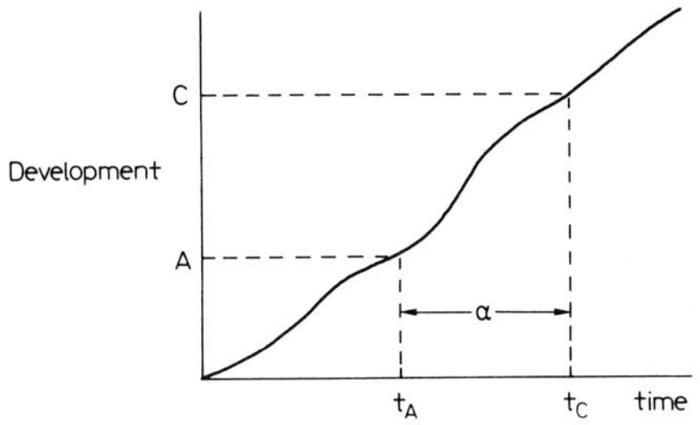

Fig. 1. Relationship between the development of a disorder and its detection by the test and the patient (see text).

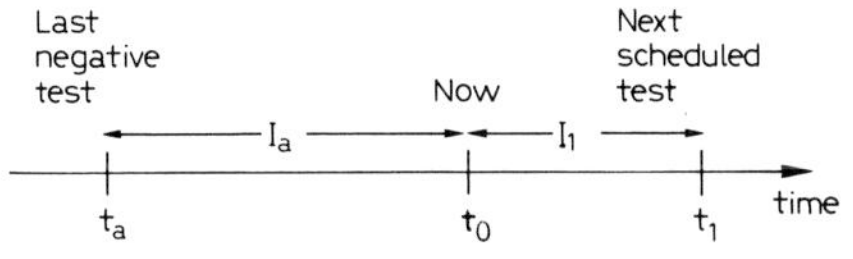

Fig. 2. Main times and events in a monitoring program (see text).

$$\{A_0^+ \mid A_a^-, C_0^+\} = \frac{\int_0^\infty [F(x + I_a) - F(x)]\, re^{-rx}\, dx}{\int_\infty^0 F(x + I_a)\, re^{-rx}\, dx}, \tag{1}$$

where I_a is the interval since the last negative test, r is the instantaneous incidence rate at which disorders are expected to occur, and F(.) is the cumulative distribution of the occult interval.

Additional equations are needed to complete the analysis. If the test performed at time t_a was negative, and the patient has no obvious signs or symptoms now (at t_0), there is a chance that the patient will develop obvious signs of the disorder before the next scheduled monitoring test, to be performed I_1 periods from now at time t_1, $\{C_1^+ \mid C_0^+, A_a^-\}$. Using reasoning similar to that given in *Eddy* [2], it can be shown that:

$$\{C_1^+ \mid C_0^-, A_a^-\} = \frac{\int_0^{I_1} F(x + I_a)\, re^{-rx}\, dx}{\int_0^\infty F(x + I_a)\, re^{-rx}\, dx}, \tag{2}$$

where $I_1 = t_1 - t_0$. By letting $t_a = t_0$, we can also use equation 2 to calculate $\{C_1^+ \mid C_0^-, A_0^-\}$. Because the time since the previous monitoring test (I_a), and the time to the next scheduled test (I_1) are variables, these equations can be used to compute the probability of detecting disorders by different methods in a program of any configuration and frequency. There is no requirement that I_a and I_1 be equal or constant.

Earliness of Detection

With equations 1 and 2 one can calculate for any monitoring frequency the probability that a disorder will be detected by the test at a particular monitoring session or will become obvious during an interval between tests. The next step is to calculate the costs and benefits of the outcomes that occur when disorders are discovered. This introduces the notion of the earliness of detection.

Figure 3 shows the life of a particular disorder as a time line, and marks two moments: the first moment it is detectable by the test (t_A), and the moment it will become obvious in the absence of monitoring (t_C). (In the figure, $T_A < T_C$, but the equations allow for the possibility that the two moments can occur in any order.) Also marked on the line are times at which monitoring tests are scheduled (denoted as 1st test, 2nd test, 3rd test, and 4th test).

Given the particular situation depicted in figure 3, the first two tests will be negative, because they are performed before the first moment of detectability (t_A). The 3rd test, however, will detect the disorder since it is performed between times t_A and t_C. Thus, the time the 3rd test is performed becomes the time designated as t_0 in figure 2.

The earliness of detection, which we designate as ε, is defined as the length of time between the moment a disorder is actually detected, by whatever means, and the moment it would have become obvious in the absence of monitoring (t_C). In this case $\varepsilon = t_C - t_0$. Notice that if the 3rd test had been scheduled later, after time t_C, the disorder would have become obvious between scheduled tests (i.e. between 2nd test and 3rd test). By definition, the earliness of detection is zero for disorders that become obvious between monitoring.

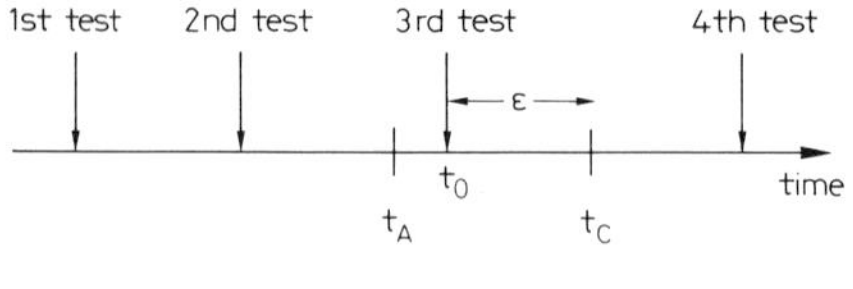

Fig. 3. Earliness of detection (see text).

The earliness of detection is a function of the effectiveness of the tests (greater effectiveness moves t_A to the left), and the frequency of screening (higher frequencies tend to move the time of actual detection to the left). Conversely, the manner in which a disorder is detected (by various tests applied at various frequencies) implies a certain earliness of detection, and it is possible to calculate the density function of the earliness of detection of disorders detected in various manners. It can be shown that:

$$\{\varepsilon \mid A_0^+, A_a^-, C_0^-\} = k[F(\varepsilon + I_a) - F(\varepsilon)]\, re^{-rx} \qquad \text{for } \varepsilon>0, \tag{3}$$

where k is a normalizing constant. Equations can be derived for the earliness of detection of disorders detected by any combination of tests in a program of any configuration.

The Outcome Function

Equations 1 and 2 are used to calculate the chance that a disorder is detected through monitoring or becomes obvious between monitorings. Equation 3 can then be used to determine how early in their natural histories these disorders are detected. The last links that connect a monitoring policy to a set of outcomes are the outcome functions, which relate the earliness with which a disorder is detected to various outcomes, such as the cost of therapy and the patient's prognosis. Any number of outcome functions can be specified, one for each outcome of interest (e.g. cost, risk of a side effect of treatment, probability of permanent damage, and so forth).

Estimation of Parameters

Three kinds of functions are required to implement the model: (1) an incidence function for the probability that a disorder will occur; (2) a density function for the occult interval of the test; and (3) the outcome functions. Each can be estimated from observable data, as described in *Eddy* [2].

Screening for Colon Cancer

The use of this computer model for monitoring gastrointestinal diseases can best be appreciated through a specific example. The questions raised by the problem of screening for colon cancer are typical of those encountered for many other conditions in gastroenterological practice.

Structure of the Colon Cancer Model

The clinical dynamics of screening for cancer of the colon are extremely complicated. Six main features were incorporated in the model to make it realistic.

(1) Mathematical formulas were written for each of the three screening tests that can be offered: digital examination of the rectal area, sigmoidoscopy, and testing for occult blood in the stool. This means that there are four ways that a malignant lesion can come to clinical attention in a screening program: through one of the three tests at a screening session, and through self-referral by the patient for symptoms in the interval between sessions. (NB: While mathematically it is possible to analyze the effects of using any or all of the screening tests in any order or frequency, in the current computer program certain simplifications were made to take advantage of actual practice patterns. In particular, since sigmoidoscopy is more expensive, more painful to the patients, and more difficult to perform, and while the test for occult blood is inexpensive (in direct costs), easily performed by the patients themselves, and readable by technicians, physicians are unlikely to do sigmoidoscopies without first doing a test for occult blood. The current computer program follows this practice and assumes that a sigmoidoscopy will always be preceded by an occult blood test and a digital examination. For example, this program can analyze the effects of performing a test for occult blood annually and a sigmoidoscopic examination biennially, but not the reverse. The computer program used to generate the results here also assumes that a digital rectal examination is always given when an occult blood test is given.)

(2) Two types of lesions were analyzed. It seems undeniable that some invasive cancers of the colon come from adenomatous polyps. It is also undeniable that some invasive lesions are not preceded by a long polyp stage but arise de novo from the crypts of the mucosa. The sigmoidoscopic examination, therefore, has two occult intervals, one for each source of cancer, that can be estimated independently. The proportion of malignant lesions that arise from adenomatous polyps is left as a parameter that can be manipulated in order to examine the implications of different assumptions about the role of these polyps. The proportion of adenomatous polyps that never proceed to a malignant stage is also a parameter of the model. (NB: It was found reasonable to simplify the computer program by having only one occult interval for the occult blood test. This was possible because data from the Minnesota Cancer Detection Center [1] and the Memorial

Sloan-Kettering Cancer Center [3] (suggest that the occult interval of this test for detecting nonmalignant polyps is very short.) The computer model must be able to analyze the impact of screening, given different assumptions about these two sources of invasive cancers.

(3) The screening tests can search different areas of the colon. A digital examination can reach 7–10cm up the rectum, depending on the technique of the examiner. A sigmoidoscope can examine the terminal 25cm of the large bowel. Occult blood tests can be positive if there is bleeding anywhere in the gastrointestinal tract. To handle these different regions, the model has, as parameters, the proportions of cancers that develop in the three main regions: the terminal 10cm, 25–10cm from the anus, and the region above 25cm from the anus. These parameters can be set to explore the implications of assuming different proportions.

(4) Lesions do not occur at the same frequency in all regions.

(5) Because incidence rates rise steadily with age, and because a sigmoidoscope can detect polyps decades before they would become symptomatic, when the same test 'looks' decades ahead it 'sees' the incidence rate of cancer in a patient decades older than the current age of that patient. It is important that the search for adenomatous polyps be based on the incidence rates, say, 5 or 10 years ahead weighted by the probability that today's polyp will turn malignant and/or cause symptoms in 5 or 10 years, for all future years (e.g. 1, 2, . . . 10, . . .) over the maximum range of premalignant polyps.

(6) The timing of the discovery of a polyp in relation to its natural history of turning malignant had to be calculated because the treatment of adenomatous polyps (by a snare, if possible) is generally less costly than the treatment of malignant polyps. Also, when a premalignant polyp is removed, the patient does not carry the diagnosis of colon cancer.

The model also adjusts for confounding factors such as the lead-time and length biases. The model is described in detail, with precise definitions of the intervals, sources for estimation of parameters, and the actual parameter values assumed, in *Eddy* [2].

Implementation

The colon cancer screening model has been programmed on a computer and can be used interactively to help clinicians and health planners estimate the consequences of different surveillance strategies. To use the program, one specifies the patient's age and sex, a relative risk factor, and the surveillance protocol that one wishes to evaluate. The user of the program also has the option of modifying a wide variety of additional parameters, to test the sensitivity of the results to changes in these parameters. Examples of parameters that can be modified include the costs of the tests, false-positive rates, the cost of diagnostic workups or treatment, the effectiveness of the tests (occult intervals), the proportions of cancers that arise from adenomatous polyps, and the proportions of cancers and adenomas that arise in various regions of the bowel.

Some Results

Costs and Effectiveness of Various Programs

This model has been used to estimate some of the cost and effectiveness measures of a variety of colon cancer screening programs. For example, values of some of the outcome measures for various screening policies for a 50-year-old, average-risk woman are shown in table I.

The first column of table I, labeled 'frequency of tests,' defines the screening program analyzed in each row. The entries give the number of years between screening tests. For example, entries '1, 2' designate a program consisting of an annual occult blood test using the Hemoccult test and a biennial sigmoidoscopy. (For brevity's sake, the term 'scope' refers to sigmoidoscopy.) The second column shows the decrease in the probability that a patient will ever be diagnosed as having colon cancer. In the absence

Table I. Colon cancer screening: cost-effectiveness measures, 50-year-old, average-risk woman [from ref. 2]

(1) Frequency of tests (e.g. every X years)		(2)	(3)	(4)	(5)
Hemoccult	Scope	Decrease in probability of diagnosis of colon cancer,.%	Increase in life expectancy, days	Decrease in lost earnings, $	Present value of program costs, $
1	1	2.82	83.83	178.17	553.14
1	2	2.66	81.37	169.38	244.69
1	3	2.55	78.84	164.48	145.08
1	4	2.43	76.71	160.34	98.60
1	5	2.29	74.54	156.25	74.09
1	never	0.09	26.69	57.66	71.86
5	5	1.65	53.27	111.14	45.09
2	4	1.68	64.80	135.06	77.63

of a screening program, a 50-year-old, average-risk woman has about a 5% chance of ever being diagnosed as having colon cancer. Since a major benefit of screening is the removal of adenomas before they become malignant, and since it is assumed in this example that 75% of all colon cancers are preceded by an adenoma, the data in this column show a major decrease in morbidity from cancer. The third column shows the increase in life expectancy in days for all women who are screened. The savings in lost earnings are given in column 4. By postponing the time of death, the screenees have a longer productive life; this is reflected by a decrease in the amount of earnings lost due to premature death. Notice that this program concerns a 50-year-old, average-risk woman, and that the expected decrease in lost earnings for a man would be considerably higher. The present value of the financial costs of the screening program (discounted at 3%) is found in column 5; the 'difference' is column 5 minus column 4.

Age to Initiate Screening

To determine the age at which screening with a sigmoidoscope should begin, let us view the problem from the standpoint of a 45-year-old, average-risk woman who is receiving an annual occult blood test and who must decide whether to begin receiving sigmoidoscopies now or wait to begin receiving this examination when she is 50 or 55 years old. Let the program consist of an annual Hemoccult test and a sigmoidoscopy every 5 years. If she never enters the program, the probability she will eventually be diagnosed as having colon cancer is about 5.06%. Table II shows the impact on some cost-effectiveness measures of starting sigmoidoscopy at various ages. This example assumes that the woman is receiving a Hemoccult test annually from age 45 on. The effect of starting this test at different ages could also be examined.

Table II. Age to initiate sigmoidoscopy: cost-effectiveness measures, 45-year-old, average-risk woman [from ref. 2]

Age to start sigmoidoscopy	Decrease in probability get cancer, %	Increase in life expectancy, days	Decrease in lost earnings, $	Present value of program costs, $
45	2.34	81.80	194.58	109.40
50	1.92	75.76	166.72	86.08
55	1.82	67.96	137.10	71.73

Table III. Effect of different assumptions about the Hemoccult false-positive rate: cost-effectiveness measures, 50-year-old, average-risk woman [from ref. 2]

False-positive rate, %	Life expectancy days	Increase in cost of differential diagnosis, $	Increase in present value of screening costs, $
1	74.54	66.81	74.09
5	75.41	330.11	337.44
10	74.25	659.23	666.63

Table IV. Effect of different polyp/cancer assumptions: cost-effectiveness measures, 50-year-old, average-risk woman [from ref. 2]

Frequency of tests (e.g. every × years)		Decrease in probability get cancer, %	Increase in life expectancy, days	Decrease in lost earnings, $	Present value of program costs, $
Hemoccult	scope				
1	1	1.19	72.84	153.09	627.27
1	5	0.59	48.15	103.01	166.79

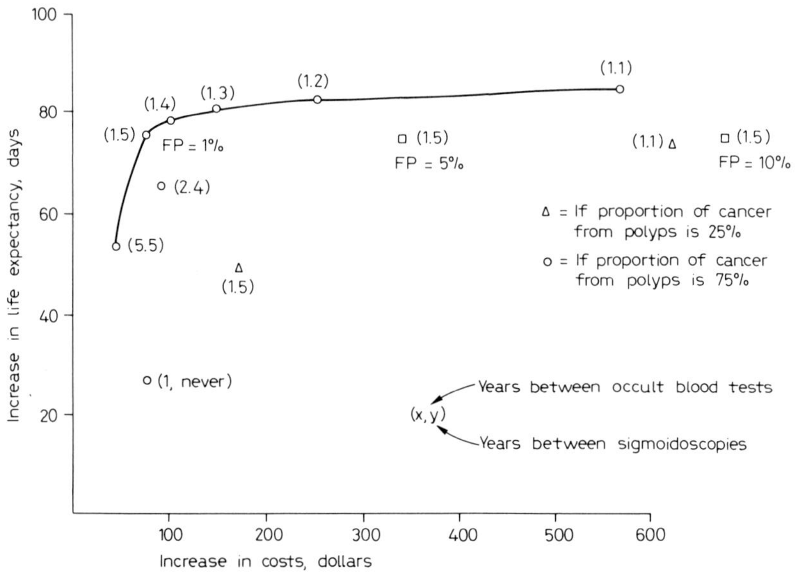

Fig. 4 Effect of assumptions about polyps and Hemoccult test false-positive rate; 50-year-old average-risk woman; increase in life expectancy versus increase in program costs for different screening policies.

Some Sensitivity Analyses

Many factors that affect the structure of a colon cancer screening program can be studied with the computer program. Consider two important ones: the false-positive rate of the occult blood test, and the proportion of malignant lesions that come from polyps.

False-Positive Rates

The false-positive rate of the occult blood test has its main effect on the risks, pain, and costs of screening. For example, when financial costs are considered, the expense of tracking down a hidden source of bleeding can be very great. In the literature, estimates of the proportion of people who do not have cancer or adenomatous polyps, but who do have positive tests, range from less than 1% to 10%. Among other things, this depends on the type of test used, the diet followed by the patient, and the circumstances of the study. There is evidence that with the Hemoccult test and with careful patient instruction, false-positive rates can be kept in the range of 0.5–2%. The importance of a low false-positive rate is shown in table III, which gives the life expectancy and present value of screening costs for a 50-year-old, average-risk woman under different assumptions about the proportion of noncancer patients who have positive Hemoccult tests. The screening program in this example is an annual Hemoccult test and a sigmoidoscopy every 5 years. The importance of the false-positive rate is obvious from this table.

The Role of Polyps

Another very important factor affecting screening is the role of adenomatous polyps in the genesis of malignant lesions. The results given above are based on the assumption that 75% of malignant lesions come from adenomatous polyps. However, there is considerable uncertainty about this number. One value of this screening theory is that we can examine the impact of different assumptions. For example, if only 25% of malignant lesions come from adenomatous polyps and 75% come directly and rapidly from the mucosa, we would expect to observe cost-effectiveness measures such as those in table IV. These results are for a 50-year-old, average-risk woman who receives (1) an annual Hemoccult (with a false-positive rate of 1%) and sigmoidoscopy, or (2) a Hemoccult annually and sigmoidoscopy every 5 years.

The changes in life expectancy and changes in program costs associated with these different assumptions about the Hemoccult false-positive rate and the role of polyps are shown in figure 4. The points marked by squares are the points associated with different false-positive rates (FP); the points marked by triangles are points generated by assuming that the proportion of cancer from polyps is 25%.

References

1 Gilbersten, V.A.: The use of screening technique for blood in the stool as a means of detecting early cancer of the bowel. Semi-annual Progress Report, End Year 6.5, January 31, 1982.

2 Eddy, D.M.: Screening for cancer: theory, analysis and design (Prentice-Hall Inc., N.J., Englewood Cliffs 1980).

3 Winawer, S.J.; Fleisher, M.; Baldwin, M.; Sherlock, P.: Current status of fecal occult blood testing in screening for colorectal cancer. Ca-A Cancer J. Clins *32*: 100–112 (1982).

D.M. Eddy, MD, PhD, Center for Health Policy Research and Education, Box GM, Duke Station, Durham, NC 27706 (USA)

Front. gastrointest. Res., vol. 7, pp. 147–185 (Karger, Basel 1984)

Computer Retrieval and Analysis of Gastroenterology Literature

Lionel M. Bernstein, Elliot R. Siegel, Charles A. Sneiderman

Lister Hill National Center for Biomedical Communications, National Library of Medicine, National Institutes of Health, Bethesda, Md., USA

Introduction

The gastroenterologist's problem in retrieving information from the published literature is not unique; it is a problem that holds for all branches of medicine, and indeed, is generic for all of science and technology. The purpose of this chapter is to briefly describe some examples of existing mechanisms that can be helpful to the searcher for gastroenterological information. This chapter is restricted to the role of computers in retrieval of information from the biomedical literature; it does not deal with the burgeoning and important uses of computers in the active decision-making processes which use that information (e.g. Caduceus, ONCOCIN).

Retrieval of the gastroenterologic literature should be considered in the context of the communication channels used by medical practitioners, educators and researchers [1, 22]. Both 'formal' and 'informal' communication are used. Formal communication is typically asymmetric, in that it normally restricts or prohibits feedback; informal communication normally encourages it. Usually, formal communication also involves preparation, and is characterized by a lack of spontaneity.

Another means useful for distinguishing between the two is that informal messages are generally transmitted via face-to-face communication channels; formal messages are typically mediated by a mechanical device interposed between the source and the intended receiver(s). An obvious exception is the telephone, as are the newer teleconferencing media that permit interactive two-way communication. Primary, secondary, and tertiary communications systems utilize both formal and informal communication channels. Primary messages are about information not previously com-

Table I. Scientific communication channels [from ref. 1]

Communications Systems	Formal	Informal
Primary	journal articles, monographs, dissertations, proceedings of meetings, reports, reprints, patents	meetings, seminars, letters, conversations
Secondary	bibliographies, listings, indexes, abstract journals, SDI services, dictionaries, catalogs, newsletters	letters, conversations
Tertiary	critical reviews, state-of-the-art surveys, review books, yearbooks, handbooks, textbooks, encyclopedias	lectures (classes), conferences, symposia letters, conversations

municated; secondary messages about primary messages which affect awareness of their existence and availability; tertiary messages about the content of other messages (table I).

The Information Explosion in Biomedicine

Over the past century the number of biomedical serials has increased steadily at a rate of about 5% per year [14]. In 1977 there were published an estimated 2,873 biomedical periodicals, constituting about one third of the estimated 8,915 total of periodicals for all of science and technology published in the USA alone. When restricted to a defined subset of 'scholarly' US publications, there were 129,000 articles published in 1,173 journals in that year [19]. From worldwide sources, there are more than 22,000 serials collected by the National Library of Medicine [14]. An additional 'explosive' effect results from an order of magnitude increase in the numerical data within articles due to automated laboratory instrumentation [25].

Increasing numbers of publications have been accompanied by increased costs. In 1977, expenditures in the USA associated with biomedical journals, books, and reports were estimated as $3 billion. This includes $428 million in costs of authoring (but not including the costs of the underlying research and development); $1,108 million publication costs; $184 million library costs, including expenditures associated with acquisition, processing, storage, abstracting, indexing, and dissemination; and $1,273 million user costs, including the economic value of time spent by biomedical researchers and educators searching for and reading the literature [19]. Were user costs of health care practitioners included, the totals would be higher. The startingly large US cost in 1977 of producing, distributing, and reading the biomedical literature is 25% of the estimated $12 billion expended for communication in all of science and technology [11]. Biomedical literature costs are projected to rise to more than $5 billion by 1985 [19]. Obviously, the costs rise greatly as one includes expenditure of biomedical communications resources in countries other than the USA.

The Uneven Quality of the Published Literature

Comments about the quantitative information overload merge with criticisms of the quality of the published literature. From many quarters have come barrages of criticism about the variable quality of the scientific and technical literature [4, 25, 27, 28, 29]. The quantitative publication overload is made much worse by these qualitative problems. Thus, it is perhaps not surprising that very much of the scientific literature is not cited, not read, not sought, and not useful. Of scientific publications, 25–50% are never cited even once [7]. A study at the British Lending Library for Science and Technology showed that in a 1-year period more than one half the collection was not consulted; that another 25% was consulted only once; and that further, from the total of 9,000 periodicals, 50% of loan requests were filled from 40, and 80%, from 900 titles [26]. At the National Library of Medicine, 300 of its, 22,000 serial titles satisfy 70% of the 200,000 interlibrary loans requested annually [5]. Of 27 million citations to 10 million science articles appearing in 24,000 journals, 50% of all citations were to articles in only 152 journals [7]. Nonetheless, whatever the deficits, publication of research results is the main and obligatory original source for knowledge that is transferred. Research results enter science only when published [28]. For the past 300 years the accretion of scientific knowledge has relied almost entirely on publication.

Awareness and understanding of current medical knowledge is essential for all practitioners in reaching the best diagnostic, prognostic and therapeutic decisions. Figure 1 schematically relates current medical know-

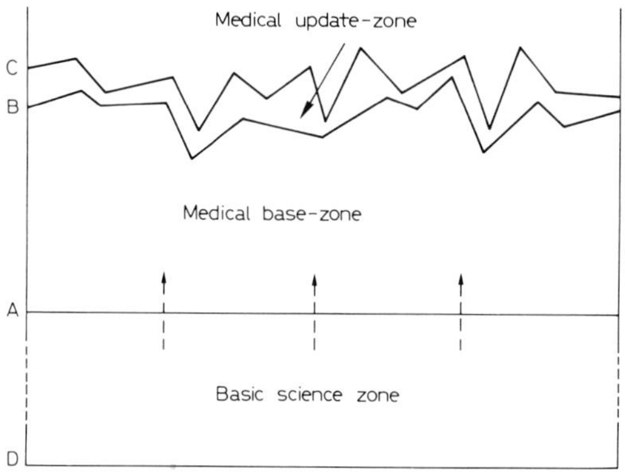

Fig. 1. The domain of medical knowledge. The medical base-zone includes that portion of underlying basic science necessary for the high-quality practice of medicine.

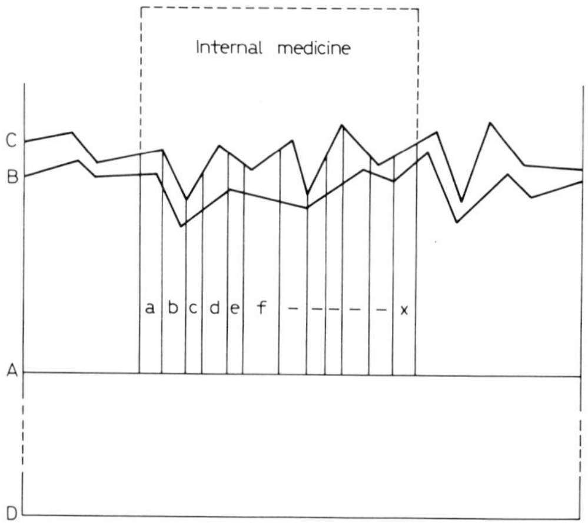

Fig. 2. The domain of internal medicine. Subspecialites of internal medicine represented by a to x encompass both medical base-zone (A-B) and medical update-zone (B-C) information.

ledge at one point in time, an increment to that current knowledge over time, and the basic science underpinnings. The medical base-zone (fig. 1 A–B) is a snapshot at one point in time of current medical knowledge necessary for the practice of medicine, and A–D is the extensive basic science knowledge upon which it is constructed. The medical base-zone includes those portions of basic science necessary for understanding and high

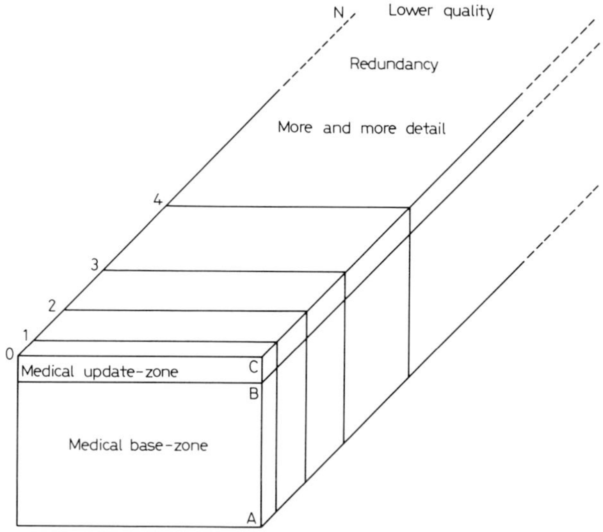

Fig. 3. Relationship of biomedical literature to the domain of medical information (see text for explanation).

quality practice of medicine. Over a period of time, there has accrued new medical knowledge (fig. 1 B–C, the medical update-zone) which becomes incorporated into a later version of the current medical base-zone.

The body of medical knowledge is somewhat arbitrarily partitioned into disciplines and fields. Internal medicine, the central core of medical practice, consists of perhaps one half of the total knowledge. In turn, it is divided into a series of complexly interrelated subspecialties (fig. 2 a–x) of which gastroenterology is one. There exist quite variable amounts and quality of information in these subdivisions. There is much overlap in the knowledge relevant to practice of the individual subspecialties of internal medicine, as well as with other major specialties such as surgery, obstetrics and gynecology, psychiatry, etc.

The well-known information explosion in biomedicine has resulted in an immense volume of published gastroenterologic and medical literature. Figure 3 adds the third dimension to characterize this volume of literature. For ease of illustration, the lines representing the boundaries of the medical knowledge zones have been straightened. The total volume of the world's published literature is area A–C multiplied by the depth O–N, a large fraction of which is redundant and, with increasing exploration, is found to contain more and more non-useful detail and lower quality information. Arbitrarily, four subsets of that immense literature are shown (0–1, 0–2, 0–3, 0–4) to emphasize that different kinds and amounts of information detail are required by different users. Different levels of detail and sophistication are needed to increase likelihood of meeting the greatly varying and differing needs of potential users [2] ranging from students to practicing subspecialists. Gastroenterology is one subset of the total. The physician needs to retrieve information from both the base – and the updating zones. The computer helps in many ways.

Approaches to Updating the Medical Literature: Current Examples

In general, the purpose of the UPDATING APPROACH is to provide selected packages of new medical information, and corrections of or additions to the older information of the medical base-zone. Use of this approach implies that the users are knowledgeable about that base-zone or will gain needed base information by other routes. To emphasize newly developed important information is, in the main, to ignore the static areas without new advances, and leads to developing bodies of information without total coherent coverage of the individual subspecialties. The huge, varied, and extensive efforts by publishers and authors to provide medical updating information attests to both the popularity and recognized need for it.

Preparing medical updating-zone information is accomplished by a mix of two methodologies – quality filtering and synthesizing. Quality filtering [6] is the selection from the mass of newly published information those pieces of particular importance, relevance and high quality. Synthesizing is the placing of the new information into context with other new and with existing older information. Review of some examples of existing systems and activities will convey the critical role of the computer in information retrieval.

The National Library of Medicine

The National Library of Medicine (NLM) is the premiere archive of the world's medical literature. Its mission has been to acquire and preserve books, periodicals, prints, films, recordings, and other library materials pertinent to medicine; organize those materials by appropriate cataloging, indexing, and bibliographical listing; and to publish and make available catalogs, indexes, and bibliographies. The NLM's bibliographic efforts began with the publication more than 100 years ago of *Index Medicus* and the *Index Catalog of the Library of the Surgeon General's Office*. The Library has had a leading role in the rapid dissemination of information. Revolutionary library technology such as photoduplication for interlibrary loans and computerized information storage and retrieval systems were pioneered by the NLM. Its current collection of 3,000,000 items provides a source of information made available to the USA and to many foreign countries.

The NLM is primarily a bibliographic resource – a transmitter rather than a producer of medical knowledge. Nonetheless, it has a crucial effect on dissemination of medical knowledge. From worldwide sources, the NLM collects 23,000 serial publications, but because of its selective indexing policy (a crucial quality filter), only about 3,000 are indexed for use. Approximately 250,000 articles are indexed annually, and more than half are accompanied by abstracts. This quality filtering process is implemented by peer expert group selection of the most appropriate journals to index.

To be useful to potential users, access to the extremely complex, multifaceted, massive biomedical literature is critical. To avoid chaos, there is required consistent, regularized, and broadly accepted common approaches to collection, classification, organization, indexing, cataloging and abstracting of that literature. This central and indispensable framework is provided to the library, information science, and health professional communities by NLM; its methods, products and services have been the framework used throughout the world for accessing and using publications in medicine and related sciences.

A major contribution to efficient and accurate retrieval of needed gastroenterologic information is made possible by the computer coupled with the time-tested indexing methods of the NLM which are the core of its Medical Literature Analysis and Retrieval System (MEDLARS). Indexing is accomplished using Medical Subject Headings (MeSH terminology), a controlled vocabulary of 14,000 designated terms which are at the heart of MEDLARS and its computerized online version, MEDLINE (and the many other NLM online data bases, see table II). Use of Boolean operators (logical 'and', 'or', and 'not') aids greatly in the computer selection of the bibliographic information sought.

Other techniques (e.g. free text and string searches) further augment the precision of retrieved information. The gastroenterologist participates in, and gains from, the broad generic capabilities of the NLM's retrieval systems. The use of the MeSH-MEDLARS indexing approach gives great

Table II. Data bases available on NLM online network

Medline (includes the next 4 items)
Index Medicus Journals
Special List Dental Journals
Special List Nursing Journals
Special List Hospital Journals
TOXLINE (Toxicology Information Online)
CHEMLINE (Chemical Dictionary Online)
RTECS (Registry of Toxic Effects of Chemical Substances, formerly the Toxic Substances List)
TDB (Toxicology Data Bank)
CATLINE (Catalog Online)
SERLINE (Serials Online)
AVLINE (Audiovisuals Online)
HEALTH PLANNING AND ADMIN (Health Planning and Administration)
HISTLINE (History of Medicine Online)
CANCERLIT (Cancer Literature)
CANCERPROJ (Cancer Research Projects)
CLINPROT (Clinical Cancer Protocols)
BIOTHICSLINE (Online File on Bioethical Topics)
EPILEPSYLINE (Online File on Epilepsy)
POPLINE (Population Information Online)

flexibility to the searcher. The basic character of a search is determined by the searcher's interest in substantive material – for example, information about a given gastroenterological disease. However, as shown in table III, there are many other attributes of information which, in the indexing process, are tagged to the pieces of information and can be used to refine the retrieval to match the user's interest more specifically. Additionally, 'explosions' of MeSH headings allows searches to include many terms related to those selected in the search strategy.

The following are of particular interest to the gastroenterologist beyond the main MEDLINE data base. This information is updated periodically, and is available in 'Fact Sheets' from the National Library of Medicine NIH, Bethesda, Md.

(1) TOXLINE (TOXicology Information OnLINE). TOXLINE is a collection of about 500,000 references from the last 5 years on published human and animal toxicity studies, effects of environmental chemicals and pollutants, and adverse drug reactions. Older material (862,000 references)

Table III. Subheadings of MeSH indexing system

Abnormalities	legislation and jurisprudence
Administration and dosage	manpower
Adverse effects	metabolism
Analogs and derivatives	methods
Analysis	microbiology
Anatomy and histology	mortality
Antagonists and inhibitors	nursing
Biosynthesis	occurrence
Blood	organization and administration
Blood supply	parasitology
Cerebrospinal fluid	pathogenicity
Chemical synthesis	pathology
Chemically induced	pharmacodynamics
Classification	physiology
Complications	physiopathology
Congential	poisoning
Cytology	prevention and control
Deficiency	psychology
Diagnosis	radiation effects
Diagnostic use	radiography
Diet therapy	radionuclide imaging
Drug effects	radiotherapy
Drug therapy	rehabilitation
Economics	secondary
Education	secretion
Embryology	standards
Enzymology	supply and distribution
Ethnology	surgery
Etiology	therapeutic use
Familial and genetic	therapy
Genetics	toxicity
Growth and development	transmission
History	transplantation
Immunology	trends
Injuries	ultrastructure
Innervation	urine
Instrumentation	utilization
Isolation and purification	veterinary

is in back files. The creation and maintenance of TOXLINE is accomplished by use of material from NLM's *Index Medicus* journals augmented by a variety of files obtained from other Federal and non-government agencies.

(2) CHEMLINE (CHEMical dictionary OnLINE). Chemical Abstracts Service contains a Registry Nomenclature File of 5.5 million chemical compounds, a subset of which is identified as the CHEMLINE data base. CHEMLINE is a file of 900,000 names for chemical substances, representing 540,000 unique compounds. CHEMLINE serves as a dictionary for chemical names and a directory for entry into TOXLINE, MEDLINE, and RTECS, and is an indispensible part of effective user entry into those data bases.

(3) Registry of Toxic Effects of Chemical Substances (RTECS). RTECS contains acute toxicity data for approximately 41,000 substances. The National Institute for Occupational Safety and Health (NIOSH) creates RTECS and the NLM puts RTECS online. This data base provides synthesized information as well as bibliographic data.

(4) Toxicology Data Bank (TDB). This online file containing chemical, pharmacologic, and toxicologic data extracted from textbooks, handbooks, criteria documents and monographs is prepared by NLM and made available online. TDB contains information and data on approximately 3,700 substances. This data base also provides synthesized information as well as bibliographic data.

(5) CATLINE (CATalog OnLINE). CATLINE contains about 462,000 references to books and serials cataloged at NLM, and provides access to authoritative cataloging information needed by medical libraries for ordering of books and journals and for providing reference and Interlibrary Loan services.

(6) AVLINE (AudioVisuals OnLINE). AVLINE contains citations to approximately 11,000 audiovisual teaching packages used in health sciences education and for continuing education of practitioners. Cataloging of audiovisuals is accomplished by NLM staff. Evaluations by content specialists in appropriate professional fields have been added to the basic bibliographic record.

(7) CANCERLIT (CANCER LITerature). CANCERLIT is a bibliographic data base on the cancer literature derived from 3,000 serials, books, and reports, and material selected from professional meeting abstracts. It contains more than 320,000 references dealing with various aspects of cancer. All references have English abstracts.

(8) CANCERPROJ (CANCER Research PROJects). CANCERPROJ contains descriptions of ongoing cancer research projects in many countries. Until recently, this online data base was prepared from research abstracts and projects maintained by the Smithsonian Scientific Information Exchange, on organization which no longer exists. A new contractor will be selected. CANCERPROJ has 9,000–10,000 new or modified research projects entered per year, and has a total of approximately 20,000 items online covering the most recent 3 year period.

(9) CLINPROT (CLINical Cancer PROTocols). CLINPROT is an online version of the National Cancer Institute's Compilation of Clinical Protocol Summaries, a hard copy publication. This data base serves as a summary of approximately 3,000 experimental protocols for cancer treatment now underway.

(10) BIOETHICSLINE (OnLINE File for BIOETHICal Topics). BIOETHICSLINE is a file of about 13,000 bibliographic references to materials on bioethical topics such as euthanasia, human experimentation and abortion. BIOETHICSLINE is produced in cooperation with the Kennedy Institute of Ethics.

The NLM offers other aids to finding the gastroenterologic literature which range from a listing of current journals in gastroenterology indexed (table IV) to publication of individual subject Literature Searches. NLM's series of Literature Searches are distributed in response to requests. These non-recurring bibliographies are selected on the basis of importance of subject matter as determined by suggestions from professional societies, NIH conferences, major new NIH research initiatives, important epidemiologic problems, suggestions from other Federal agencies, and from many of the reader constituencies. Primary emphasis is placed on clinical subjects for clinical target audiences. The bibliographies contain references to recent articles selected from the MEDLINE data base. Search strategies aim for a maximum of 300 citations per Literature Search. Their purpose is to provide bibliographies of the current literature that would be of wide interest

Table IV. Gastroenterology journals indexed by NLM

Acta gastroenterologica belgica (Bruxelles)	Gut (London)
Acta gastroenterologica Latinoamericana (Buenos Aires)	Hepato-gastroenterology (Stuttgart)
American Journal of Gastroenterology (New York)	Hepatology (American Association for Study of Liver Disease) (Baltimore)
American Journal of Proctology Gastroenterology and Colon and Rectal Surgery (Georgetown, Conn.)	Journal of Clinical Gastroenterology (New York)
Arquivos de Gastroenterologia (Sao Paulo)	Leber, Magen, Darm (Baden-Baden)
Ceskoslovenska Gastroenterologie A Vyziva (Praha)	Medicine et Chirurgie Digestives (Paris)
Clinics in Gastroenterology (London)	Minerva Dietologica E Gastroenterologica (Torino)
Deutsche Zeitschrift für Verdauungs- und Stoffwechselkrankheiten (Leipzig)	Nippon Shokakibyo Gakkai Zasshi, Japanese Journal of Gastroenterology (Tokyo)
Digestion (Basel)	Peptides (Fayetteville, N.Y.)
Digestive Diseases and Sciences (New York)	Progress in Liver Disease (New York)
Diseases of the Colon and Rectum (Philadelphia)	Recent Avances in Gastroenterology (Edinburgh)
Endoscopy (Stuttgart)	Regulatory Peptides (Amsterdam)
Frontiers of Gastrointestinal Research (Basel)	Revista Espanola de las Enfermedades del Aparato Digestivo (Madrid)
Gastroenterologia Japonica (Tokyo)	Revista de Gastroenterologia de Mexico (Mexico)
Gastroenterologie Clinique et Biologique (Paris)	Scandinavian Journal of Gastroenterology (Oslo)
Gastroenterology (Baltimore)	Scandinavian Journal of Gastroenterology, Supplement (Oslo)
Gastrointestinal Endoscopy (Denver, Colo.)	Tijdschrift voor Gastro-Enterologie (Antwerpen)
Gastrointestinal Radiology (Berlin)	Zeitschrift für Gastroenterologie (München)
Gen (Caracas)	Zeitschrift für Gastroenterologie Verhandlungsband (München)

to the user communities, thereby minimizing the numbers of individual searches on the same subject by individual users. There have been approximately 500 such Literature Searches produced over the past 15 years, many of which are relevant to the field of gastroenterology.

Of great importance to gastroenterology (as well as to other specialties of medicine) are the continuing improvements in the NLM's retrieval systems. The NLM has had, and can expect to continue to have, active liaisons with professional organizations through which there is identified need for new indexing concepts and terminology. Thus, the MEDLARS system continuously evolves to accommodate and include new medical advances. Significant technical advances have been made on NLM's retrieval capabilities and more can be expected. Research by NLM staff as well as by industry and university based researchers has led to new systems that will be *much more cordial* to users, and will have simplicity of use with the potential for overcoming computer terminal reluctance of most audiences. Continuing improvement in retrieval capabilities can be expected.

Excerpta Medica

Excerpta Medica is an information retrieval service that indexes and abstracts biomedical and clinical literature. A major emphasis is placed on professional abstracting by practicing physicians. 60% of its records include abstracts. Excerpta Medica publishes two indexes of bibliographic references to the Drug Literature, 43 journals containing abstracts of articles published in the primary journal literature and six core journals containing abstracts for discrete clinical specialties from the 43 abstract journals. Annually, 400,000 articles from 35,000 journals are screened and 240,000 articles per year (150,000 with abstracts) are included in the 43 specialty journals. Excerpta Medica products are directed to clinicians and research scientists. Two million records have been entered into Excerpta Medica since 1967; updating occurs every 2 months.

Excerpta Medica abstract journals include one series on internal medicine as well as one series for each of almost all the subspecialties of medicine, including gastroenterology (table V). Cumulative indexes are published in the individual hard copy columes. Access to both text of abstracts and the indexes is available online through DIALOG. The Excerpta Medica selection of articles and their abstracting by physicians constitutes another very large quality filtering effort, but one which differs in methodology from that of the National Library of Medicine. The two systems have some overlap in the journals and individual articles covered (approximately 25–30%), but overall offer distinctly different responses to subject search inquiries. A further important difference is the wide array of hard copy medical texts produced and published by Excerpta Medica.

Institute for Scientific Information

The Institute for Scientific Information (ISI) provides an interesting and wide range of information services, including some very innovative in character. ISI provides a comprehensive information discovery and re-

Table V. Excerpta Medica abstract journals

Anatomy, Anthropology, Embryology and Histology
Anesthesiology
Arthritis and Rheumatism
Biophysics, Bio-engineering and Medical Instrumentation
Cancer
Cardiovascular Diseases and Cardiovascular Surgery
Chest Diseases, Thoracic Surgery and Tuberculosis
Clinical Biochemistry
Dermatology and Venerology
Developmental Biology and Teratology
Drug Dependence
Endocrinology
Environmental Health and Pollution Control
Epilepsy
Forensic Science Abstracts
Gastroenterology
General Pathology and Pathological Anatomy
Gerontology and Geriatrics
Health Economics and Hospital Management
Hematology
Human Genetics
Immunology, Serology and Transplantation
Internal Medicine
Leprosy and Related Subjects
Microbiology: Bacteriology, Mycology and Parasitology
Neurology and Neurosurgery
Nuclear Medicine
Obstetrics and Gynecology
Occupational Health and Industrial Medicine
Ophthalmology
Orthopedic Surgery
Oto-, Rhino-, Laryngology
Pediatrics and Pediatric Surgery
Pharmacology and Toxicology
Physiology
Plastic Surgery
Psychiatry
Public Health, Social Medicine and Hygiene
Radiology
Rehabilitation and Physical Medicine
Surgery
Urology and Nephrology
Virology

trieval system including weekly alert bulletins (Current Contents); a selective dissemination and document provision service; and two large interdisciplinary data bases, the Science Citation Index (online as SCISEARCH), and Social Science Citation Index (online as Social SCISEARCH).

Commonly known is *Current Contents*, published sets of replicas of the tables of contents of current journal issues, distributed by subscription. The result is quick and convenient browsing of (only the) titles and authors of newly published work. More sophisticated is the publication of Science Citation Index (SCI) and Social Science Citation Index (SSCI). SCI classifies and groups articles on the basis of their citing of specific documents within the 2,600 journals (and 3,000,000 records) in the SCI data base. This serves as a new kind of indexing – the classification of content of articles on the basis of authors' judgements of what literature is relevant to their writings. Thus, this unique searching capability links authors and their areas of work in a new way. SCI/SSCI data also have been used by some as measures of the usefulness and impact of scientific publications, and the 'quality' of the underlying scientific work. SCI does provide new insights in tracing a subject content area over time, and for understanding the social relationships in science. Journal Citation Reports provides similar citation data for individual journal titles rather than for individual journal articles.

Co-citation analysis builds on the basic citation analysis data to provide greatly more intricate and sophisticated entries to the scientific literature. Co-citation clustering is a method used to identify a group of highly cited *and* closely related papers which together form the core of the significant work in a given substantive area. The act of co-citing papers – that is, when each of a set of papers cites the same combination of other papers – establishes similarity of interest of the citing papers. When applied to the very recent literature, the method is useful in identifying and characterizing areas of intense research activity called new 'Research Fronts'. This new capability derives from the ISI/BIOMED SEARCH data base. Perusing titles of these identified and described Research Fronts will reveal cores of articles in new subfields some of which are relevant to the subspecialty of gastroenterology.

Biosciences Information Service

The Biosciences Information Service covers basic research in the life sciences including agriculture, biochemistry, bioengineering, biophysics, ecology, experimental medicine, microbiology, and pharmacology. Approximately 9,000 scientific journals are screened, as well as are books, monographs, meetings and conference proceedings, semi-popular journals, research communications, and symposia. Three million records from 1969 to the present are available online on BIOSIS. Approximately 23,500 records are added monthly. BIOSIS Previews is the bibliographic data base corresponding to the printed versions of Biologic Abstracts (BA) and Biological Abstracts (RRM).

Chemical Abstracts Service

Chemical Abstracts (CA) provides international coverage of the chemical literature from more than 14,000 scientific and technical journals, as well as conference proceedings, congresses and symposia, technical reports, dissertations, new books, announcements, and patents from 26 countries. Approximately one third of the literature is biochemical. The indexes to CA are numerous and complex. The CA SEARCH online data base contains bibliographic data, keyword phrases, and index entries for all documents covered by Chemical Abstracts Service. It contains about 5,000,000 records covering 1967 to the present. CA SEARCH is an expanded data base which contains the basic bibliographic information appearing in the printed Chemical Abstracts, and the CASIA file, which contains CA General Subject Headings from a controlled vocabulary and the CAS Registry Numbers, a unique number assigned to each specific chemical compound. Additional uncontrolled vocabulary terms and cross-referenced CA General Subject Headings are also included.

Information Retrieval Limited

Information Retrieval Limited (IRL) does abstracting in 15 discrete areas of biology and medical sciences. It thoroughly covers journals, books, conference proceedings, reports, patents, and other literature in its specific areas. IRL screens 5,500 periodicals, contains 440,000 records entered since January 1978, adds 110,000 records per year and is updated weekly. It provides full abstracts in English. Indexing and abstracting are done by university graduates in the life sciences.

Psychological Abstracts

Psychological Abstracts, with its online version PSYCINFO, is prepared by the American Psychological Association. PSYCINFO covers the world's literature in psychology and related disciplines in the behavioral sciences. Over 900 periodicals and 1,500 books, technical reports, and monographs are scanned each year to provide coverage of original research, reviews, discussion, theory, conference reports, panel discussions, case studies, and descriptions of apparatus. It includes both human and animal aspects in: animal psychology; applied psychology; communication and language; cultural influences and social issues; developmental psychology; education; neurology and physiology; perception and motor performance; personality; physical and psychological disorders; psychometrics and statistics; treatment and prevention; and personnel and professional issues. It covers the psychology and behavior of groups and organizations in addition to that of individuals. PSYCINFO contains about 350,000 citations from 1967 to the present.

Other Updating Publications

A very large number and wide variety of other publications exist to provide updating information. Currently, the support of these by computer is in the publication process for some (e.g. providing computer tapes of text for camera ready photocomposition copy) and for usual bibliographic location of books, journals and some reports. Just as hard copy paper publication of bibliographic information (e.g. *Index Medicus*) preceded and was later extended to much more versatile online bibliographic tools (e.g. MEDLINE), it will be of interest over the next several years to watch the extent to which electronic publishing made possible by new computer and communications technologies complements and/or displaces current paper publications. The following examples are presented to remind the gastroenterologist of how extensive are the efforts to provide updating information, and to emphasize the interrelationships with other fields of medicine.

Year Books of Medicine, Surgery, etc. A series of 25 annual publications offered by the Year Book Publishers is an important example mainly of quality filtering of the medical literature, combined with small components of synthesis and some linkages to the medical base-zone (fig. 4). These 25 annual publications cover many of the specialties and subspecialties of medicine and surgery (see table VI). In the aggregate, 200,000 volumes are sold annually, attesting to the success of this approach in serving some of the information updating needs of large numbers of physicians. This private sector effort has obtained the cooperation of large numbers of medical experts to select from the mass of new journal articles a subset of those which are important to their respective disciplines because of new, relevant and high-quality information. In the Year Books it is stated that

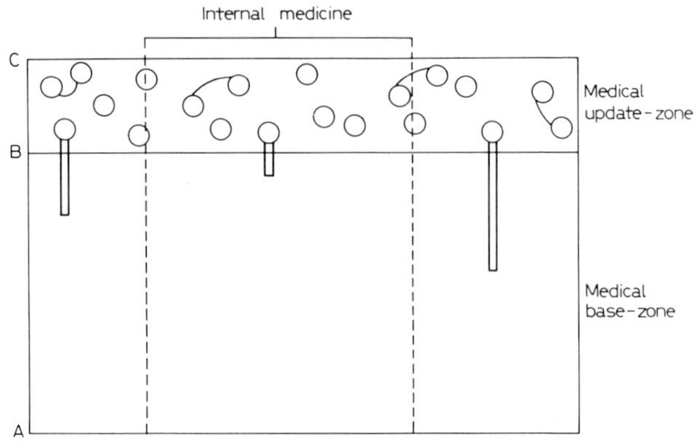

Fig. 4. Information covered by Yearbooks. Pieces of quality filtered new information are linked to some extent to other new and older information. Some synthesis is offered. There is not comprehensive coverage of any individual field.

Table VI. The 1981 year books

Anesthesia	Nuclear Medicine
Cancer	Obstetrics and Gynecology
Cardiology	Ophthalmology
Clinical Pharmacy	Orthopedics
Dentistry	Otolaryngology
Dermatology	Pathology and Clinical Pathology
Diagnostic Radiology	Pediatrics
Drug Therapy	Plastic and Reconstructuve Surgery
Emergency Medicine	Psychiatry and Applied Mental Health
Endocrinology	Sports Medicine
Family Practice	Surgery
Medicine	Urology
Neurology and Neurosurgery	

the material is selected by editors who critically review more than 500,000 journal articles each year. Each author-editor is allotted a specified amount of space or number of articles for each year's volume. Each article selected is described, usually in detail considerably greater than in the usual bibliographic abstract, but with much condensation from the journal article's actual length. Inclusion of selected figures and tables augments fidelity of reporting. For many articles the author-editor offers a brief commentary or synthesized view of the reported work and how it is linked to the medical base-zone information.

The quantity of coverage of disciplines or fields is quite variable. For example, the 1981 Year Book of Medicine includes seven sections, on Infections; Chest; Blood and Blood-Forming Organs; Heart and Blood Vessels; Digestive System; Metabolism; and Kidney, Water, and Electrolytes. Numbers of articles for each of those sections ranges from 49 to 61 – much less than for those subjects which have an entire dedicated volume – such as the 1981 Year Book of Cardiology which contains 304 articles.

The list of subjects covered by the Year Books (table VI) suggests retrieval problems that are commonplace and pervasive in all medical literature systems – problems of duplication, overlap, and gaps of the subject matter covered. An analysis of several *1981* Year Book volumes illustrates this. There is a Year Book of Cardiology, but there also are sections of cardiology within several other Year Books:

		Number of articles reported
Year Book of Cardiology		304
Chapter:	Heart and Blood Vessels in YB of Medicine	61
Chapters:	Cardiac and Vascular Disease of YB of Surgery	47
Chapter:	Heart and Blood Vessels in YB of Pediatrics	16
Chapter:	Angiography in YB of Radiology	39
Chapter:	Cardiovascular Diseases in YB of Drug Therapy	69

A detailed analysis of the articles selected reveals that the patterns of journals cited are grossly different and that there is indeed very little overlap of individual citations. Only a few of the cardiology articles are reported in more than one of these year books. Thus, a physician interested in cardiology who reads only the Year Book of Cardiology will miss much important new and relevant cardiology information selected by the experts in these other fields; and the physician who reads only the Year Book of Medicine is missing a very large fraction of the cardiology literature deemed as new and important by the quality filtering activities of the Year Book author-editors.

A brief analysis of Year Book articles in the subspecialty of gastroenterology reveals a similar pattern: the different Year Books sample different proportions or mixes of journal titles, and there is little duplication of reports on the same gastroenterology articles in the various specialty volumes.

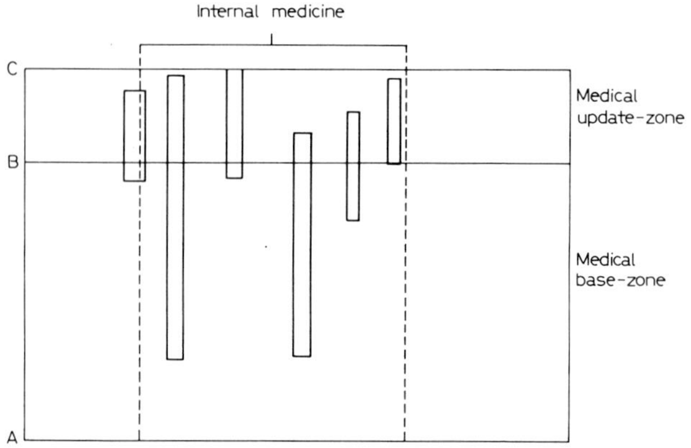

Fig. 5. Information covered by MKSAP syllabus. Synthesized summaries of quality filtered new information put in context with older base information. There is not comprehensive coverage of all of internal medicine.

The MKSAP Syllabus. The Medical Knowledge Self Assessment Program (MKSAP) of the American College of Physicians (ACP) includes the assembly and publication every few years of a syllabus containing important recent information in the subspecialties of medicine. The syllabus combines quality filtration of the literature (and other sources of information) with synthesis. Through a series of committees of experts of the ACP, brief synthesized summaries are presented for those areas deemed to have had the most significant advances since the prior MKSAP syllabus. As shown in figure 5, these syntheses present the new information in contextual connection with the medical base-zone, but their total content does not cover coherently the entire domain of internal medicine. Gastroenterology is one of the subspecialties of medicine covered.

That the latest MKSAP syllabus sold 44,000 copies attests both to the desire of physicians to obtain current information and to the users' perception of this as a successful excellent collegial effort to quality filter and synthesize recent advances in internal medicine. Of special value is the authoritativeness and credibility for a wide audience of users which derives from the consensus on content of MKSAP reached by the committees of experts.

Annual Reviews. Annual and other recurring reviews of the medical literature abound. They vary widely in the mix of quality filtration and synthesis. Their purposes are to identify new important advances, and to interpret them in the light of preexisting medical knowledge. Individual annual reviews do not cover an entire field or sub-field of interest – they do not constitute a total coherent presentation of a complete body of knowledge as is done by classical large textbooks.

The extent to which such publications are available in medicine is suggested in rough terms by searches of English language entries in SERLINE and CATLINE. SERLINE (SERials OnLINE) is the NLM's bibliographic file of 34,000 serial titles (that is, recurring publications), which are cataloged because they are in medicine or related fields. There are 449 open serial titles which contain the words 'Review' or 'Reviews'. There are 53 serial titles which contain the words 'Annual' *and* 'Reviews'. CATLINE (CATalog OnLine) is NLM's bibliographic file on 210,000 books and serials cataloged at NLM since 1965. A search of CATLINE revealed 1818 entries with the word 'Annual'; and 2,301 titles with the word 'Review' in the titles. These are minimal estimates of review publications because for each of the subspecialties there are many other published recurring and non-recurring books that are review in nature, but contain substantive titles: examples are *Medical Clinics of North America, Clinics in Gastroenterology, Progress in Liver Disease*, etc. Recent new efforts at quality filtering and synthesizing new information in gastroenterology are *Liver Annual* and *Gastroenterology Annual*. Further enumeration is not needed to affirm the extensive scope of such 'review' efforts.

Miscellaneous Efforts. Through free or subscription newsletters, brief one time state-of-art reviews, controlled circulation journal giveaways, professional service notifications, and a wide variety of other means, the health care provider is offered updating information by private-for-profit information science and promotional companies, pharmaceutical firms, professional societies, governmental health agencies, and many other sources. The *Medical Letter on Drugs and Therapeutics* is an example of a publication bringing recent information on drugs to 110,00 paying subscribers. *Viewpoints on Digestive Diseases* is a series of compact synthesized and up-to-date summaries of single important gastroenterologic subjects which is published and distributed by the American Gastroenterological Association.

Summary

Access to the vast array of updating information is supported by bibliographic tools offered through many organizations. Data bases such as those on the computers of the NLM, Excerpta Medica, and ISI can be accessed online via commercial electronic networks (e.g. Tymnet or Telenet), and via network vendors (such as BRS, SDC, and Lockheed). Document distribution of identified items is facilitated by the NLM's Regional Medical Library network. Mostly, the above systems are directed toward many broad fields; the specialty interests of gastroenterology are subsumed by their scope. Much of information retrieval in gastroenterology will be accomplished by the specific searching and application of approaches that are generic to the broader fields of biomedicine and science.

Medical Base-Zone Information

The above descriptions are glimpses of the vast amounts of both quality filtered and synthesized recent medical literature that are available. Obviously, also of great importance is access to base-zone information literature which consists of both recent syntheses of fields (e.g. standard textbooks of medicine and its subfields, monographs, etc.), as well as the 'updating literature of past times'.

Textbooks are very important synthesis efforts. The synthesizing process is designed to present to readers a coherent view of a field in a highly efficient organized and condensed form, which analyzes and contains only the most important, relevant, and high quality work, and which reduces redundancy of information to a minimum. It makes possible reasonable understanding of multiple fields by individuals which would simply not be possible were each individual required to read the mass of underlying primary literature and individually perform the intellectual synthesis. Textbooks and other tertiary literature have been a major mode by which large numbers of generalists and practitioners have gained understanding of whole fields.

There are many representations of the underlying base of knowledge in gastroenterlogy in the most recent editions of the leading broad textbooks in the field. Through a process of interest and self-selection plus selection by private sector publishers, several leading experts have assembled textual representations of the field of gastroenterology which vary in size and complexity. On most matters, authors agree on the state of knowledge; on many, they differ. Because there are many texts in gastroenterology, there are indeed many representations of the field. None is absolute – none is 'THE' field of gastroenterology. Texts are selected to meet the quite variable individual needs of the users. Thus, individual user preferences select between long and short texts; single versus multiple authors; clinical versus basic science orientations; readable homilies versus reference works; etc. There is no need here to array the titles of the large number of available texts on general gastroenterology and liver disease.

The total gastroenterologic information available, in its full detail, with its great redundancy, with its extensions into vast basic science arenas, and with its linkages to other fields of medicine – quantitatively adds up to several hundred-fold the amount of pages in any core of selected gastroenterologic textbooks. But a critical virtue of such textbooks is the enormous reduction of the vast literature that the authors have accomplished by quality filtration and synthesis – while retaining through bibliographic references, the links to that vast primary literature which awaits exploration by those who wish more. In practical terms, the leading successful textbooks do represent the essential underlying information needed for the practice of gastroenterology, along with an amount of the underlying basic sciences whose understanding is necessary for that practice. Clearly book knowledge is not itself being equated to successful high quality practice; clinical decision-making involves many other skills and behaviors. Rather, knowledge of the information in medical texts, as discussed here, should be thought of as necessary, but not in itself sufficient for good practice. Computerized catalogs (e.g. CATLINE) are routinely used as bibliographic tools to locate desired texts.

Bibliometric Research Related to the NLM's Knowledge Base Research Program

Conventional bibliographic data bases and document dissemination services have been a significant factor in information transfer to the research scientist and educator, who are heavy users of formal communication channels. However, such systems are generally inefficient transfer mechanisms for the busy health practitioner who frequently lacks the time necessary to access the formal literature and the expertise necessary to process adequately the massive amount of information likely to be available on any given patient management problem [2, 10]. Studies have found that the health practitioner places a good deal of emphasis on informal communication channels, including consultation with influential and knowledgeable colleagues [22]. In theory, these informal communication transactions trade on the colleague's ability to (1) keep abreast of new information, (2) to select, review, and synthesize from the mass of available infor-

1 2 3 4 5 6 7

881H Vertical transmission of hepatitis to neonates

882 Vertical transmission of hepatitis B virus refers to transmission occurring from mother to infant. High rates of neonatal infection occur when the mother has acute type B hepatitis near delivery, but hepatitis B in the first and second trimester is associated with a low rate of transmission. Variable rates of neonatal infection occur when the mother is an HBsAg carrier. Presence of HBeAg in the mother's serum is a positive predictor and anti-HBe is a negative predictor of vertical transmission of HBV. It is likely that some newborns are infected during the birth process and some are infected in utero. Breast milk may contain HBsAg, but its role in transmission is doubtful. Infected neonates are likely to become carriers of HBsAg and have variable transaminase elevations and histological evidence of persistent hepatitis. Vertical transmission of non-A, non-B hepatitis has been described, but type A hepatitis has not been implicated.

883 Investigation of groups of maternal HBsAg carriers discovered by screening showed vertical transmission to the infants varying from 0 to 70 percent (ref. 971, 966, 1007, 828, 45, 3950). Such differences have been attributed to relative infectivity of the mother's blood as manifested by the presence of HBeAg, HBV-specific DNA polymerase, or the presence of DNA-containing hepatitis B virions.

884 In epidemiologic studies in the small South Pacific island of Santa Cruz, clustering of HBsAg and anti-HBs positive children only in families with an HBsAg positive mother suggests vertical transmission (ref. 704).

885 Seventy percent (19 of 27) of babies became HBV infected when maternal hepatitis occurred in the third trimester or in the first two postpartum months in contrast to 6 percent (1 of 16) babies if the maternal hepatitis occurred in the first or second trimester (ref. 971).

886 In order to determine the relationship between HBeAg reactivity of HBsAg carrier mothers and the frequency with which they transmit HBV infection to their offspring, 62 babies born to carrier mothers in Taiwan were followed for an average of 5 months postpartum. Presence of HBeAg was determined by agar gel diffusion and counterelectrophoresis. Sera from 20 of the 62 mothers studied, or 32 percent, were HBeAg positive; only one woman was found to be positive for anti-HBe. Eighty-five percent of the babies born to HBeAg positive mothers became HBsAg carriers, in contrast to only 31 percent carriers among babies born to HBeAg negative mothers. Presence of HBeAg in mothers' sera closely correlated with CF titers of circulating HBsAg: the geometric mean CF titer of surface antigen in mothers HBeAg positive was 1:69 compared with 1:9 titer in HBeAg negative mothers. Both reactivity for HBeAg and high CF titers of HBsAg were found to be equally good predictors of vertical transmission (ref. 87).

887 Two anti-HBe positive mothers (one acutely ill) gave birth to babies in whom HBsAg-positive disease developed. One infant cleared HBsAg with the development of anti-HBs. The clearance of HBsAg among infected infants is unusual (ref. 362, 967, 364).

888 Transplacental infection occurs. In one case the mother developed hepatitis at six months gestation; became antigen negative before delivery; yet the cord blood was positive and the baby has been HBsAg positive since birth. This represents in utero infection. The antigen in the cord blood was produced by the infected neonate rather than by the mother (ref. 971).

889 A sample of cord blood positive for HBsAg by RIA was examined for the presence of Dane particles; several typical double-shelled particles were observed. This finding would suggest that there is no placental barrier to complete Dane particles (ref. 129).

890 Two children born of ceasarean section to mothers with severe hepatitis, and separated immediately from their mothers, still developed acute hepatitis. In neither case was HBsAg found in cord blood, amniotic fluid or placenta, yet both children developed antigenemia at 50 and 60 days of age (ref. 379).

362. Gerety, RJ, Hoofnagel, JH, Markenson, JA, et al.: Exposure to hepatitis B virus and development of the chronic HG Ag carrierstate in children. J Pediatr, 84:661, 1974.

364. Gerety, RJ: Letter: Maternal Transmission of hepatitis B. N Engl J Med, 295:170-1, 1976.

967. Schweitzer, IL, Dunn, AG, Peters, RL, et al.: Viral hepatitis B in neonates and infants. Am J Med, 55:762, 1973.

Fig. 6. Sample excerpt from HKB.

mation that which is important and relevant, and (3) to provide the needed information at a level of detail, and in a time frame that is responsive to the questioner's information needs.

In reality, however, not every health practitioner has access to an appropriate array of influential and knowledgeable colleagues, nor do all such colleagues necessarily possess equivalent abilities to perform this needed information transfer function. An idealized scenario would envision such an information resource to be uniformly and consistently available to all health practitioners at an acceptable cost. The NLM's Knowledge Base Research Program has been developed to address this method of transfer of information. The early goals of this research called for the assembly of a comprehensive body of information that would contain substantive information relevant to a wide variety of information needs (rather than bibliographic citations only); would provide information that is both current and the consensus of experts; would be immediately responsive to inquiries (online access), and would provide access to variable levels of data supporting the substantive information, including citations to primary publications for more detailed study if desired.

The initial prototype effort centered on the development of a full-text data base in the field of viral hepatitis. Research and development on the hepatitis knowledge base (HKB) prototype information transfer system is described in detail in a special supplement to the *Annals of Internal Medicine* [2] which also contains an abridged version of the HKB contents [26]. A brief overview of the HKB experiment is presented below.

A key decision in the design of the HKB was the determination to create a hierarchial, full-text data base in which are arrayed three types of information: *headings and subheadings* denoting discrete sections within the customary categorial groupings of definition, etiology, epidemiology, classification, treatment and prevention; *synthesis statement* containing succinct summaries of the current state-of-knowledge for each heading, these being derived by consensus of a panel of subject matter experts; and *data elements*, extracts from the clinical and experimental research literature – containing data and bibliographic citations, all of which are intended to serve as an authority base for the assertions made in the synthesis statements. An example of HKB text, illustrating a heading ('Vertical Transmission of Hepatitis to Neonates'), the accompanying synthesis statement, and several supporting data elements is shown in figure 6.

The initial draft version of the HKB was produced by a single individual utilizing existing viral hepatitis syntheses in the form of a major textbook chapter and some 40 review articles [15, 17, 18]. This text was subjected to validation and updating by a panel of prominent experts in the field of viral hepatitis. The HKB contents are intended to reflect a consensus view of the biomedical literature as determined by this group. Selection of newly published materials for updating purposes is largely dependent upon a core set of 18 journals identified by means of citation analysis of references cited in early versions of the HKB. (A detailed discussion of these methods is an important focus of this chapter.) Individual and group communications among the geographically dispersed members of the expert panel and the NLM's Lister Hill Center staff, including the conduct of consensus development discussions, is accomplished by means of the Electronic Information Exchange System (EIES, New Jersey Institute of Technology, Newark, N.J.), a computer-based messaging and conferencing system specifically developed to support scientific communities [9]. An Eclipse c/330 minicomputer (Data General Corp, Westborough, Mass.), utilizing the MUMPS/MIIS operating system (MEDITECH, Cambridge, Mass.), is utilized for HKB text storage and maintenance. Experimental remote online searching of the HKB contents – the principal mode of user access, is performed with the HP2648A graphics terminal (Hewlett Packard Corp., Palo Alto, Calif.) via the TELENET telecommunication network (General Telephone and Electronics Corp., McClean, Va.).

A formative evaluation of the methods utilized in the development of the HKB, as well as a limited field test of the online access system, has been carried out [20]. Results of the evaluation support the conclusion that the HKB has met the original objectives of creating a mechanism which could improve information transfer to the health practitioner community, and can serve as a model for further experimentation in other content domains. Significant enhancement of the online access system, provided by a natural language free-text search capability – a major recommendation of the evaluation report – has recently been implemented for experimental use.

As the knowledge base concept has evolved and matured, progressively greater emphasis has been placed on the fundamental research issues involving the computer-based representation of knowledge. Nevertheless, there still remains the need to identify and select from the universe of biomedical literature that which is to be acquired, evaluated, and synthesized in the course of constructing baseline text and updating that content over time. The remainder of this chapter is devoted to a discussion of the previously reported methods and strategies of quality filtration first utilized in the construction and initial updating of the HKB [2, 23] and the more recent efforts employed in connection with work on the domain of peptic ulcer disease [23].

The Hepatitis Knowledge Base Literature. In attempting to construct the initial HKB synthesis, a need for quality filters quickly became apparent. A MEDLINE search of 3,000 citations to serials (out of 22,000 potentially available) yielded a staggering 16,000 English language postings on viral hepatitis for the immediately preceding 10-year period. Reading this many articles was impractical for constructing a synthesis. After several false starts, the notion of using existing syntheses of the viral hepatitis literature was settled on as a basis for constructing the text. Experts in the field were consistent in their recommendations of a newly published text on liver disease, which contained an excellent chapter on viral hepatitis [15]. The complete proceedings of a then recently held National Academy of Sciences Symposium on Viral Hepatitis were also fortunately available [17, 18]. Together, the text book chapter and the 40 symposium reviews served as the quality filter of the viral hepatitis literature.

Why are review articles good quality filters? Drawing on personal knowledge and experience, authors of review articles select from the mass of published literature that which is of highest quality and most relevant. In a good review the reader is presented with a highly organized, concise analytic summary; and because of space limitations, the author is forced to limit the number and redundancy of the bibliographic citations. *Pao* [16] and *Herring* [8] have both discussed the utility of using review articles as a quality filter mechanism.

Over a 6-month period, selected segments of the review articles were literally cut and pasted into a single body of information – a synthesis of existing syntheses. This initial version was then distributed to a ten-member panel of nationally prominent viral hepatitis experts who were asked to evaluate the synthesis and to propose additions, deletions, and modifications. Overall, the experts judged the content to be accurate and of high quality. The EIES computer conferencing system was used as the principal medium of communication linking the geographically dispersed experts with one another and with the Lister Hill Center staff [13]. Use of this teleconferencing medium also afforded the opportunity to conduct consensus development discussions independent of the constraints of space and time imposed by efforts to convene face-to-face group meetings [21].

Since the text synthesis was constucted from published reviews, the content was approximately 2.5 years out of date. A MEDLINE search

Table VII. Journal Citation Analysis (n = 575) of 1970–1975 articles referenced in initial Hepatitis Knowledge Base synthesis

Journal (n = 78)	Articles	
	number	cumulative percent
Lancet	84	15
New Engl. J. Med.	58	25
J. Am. med. Ass.	44	32
J. infect. Dis.	43	40
J. Virol.	40	47
Am. J. Epidemiol.	26	51
Gastroenterology	24	56
Proc. Soc. exp. Biol. Med.	18	59
Ann. intern. Med.	17	62
Science	16	64
Am. J. Dis. Child.	14	67
Nature, Lond.	13	69
J. Immun.	11	71
J. exp. Med.	10	73
Vox Sang.	10	74
Archs intern. Med.	9	76
Scand. J. infect. Dis.	9	78
Br. med. J.	8	79
Am. J. Med.	6	80
Can. med. Ass. J.	6	81
Intervirology	6	82
Proc. natn. Acad. Sci. USA	6	83
Am. J. Path.	5	84
Pathol. Microbiol.	5	85
Others	87	100

yielded 5,700 articles published on the subject of viral hepatitis during the intervening period. A mechanism was needed to select from among these the new and important literature and to establish a mechanism to identify prospectively new information for future content updates. Indirectly, the quality filter function of the text book chapter and the 40 review articles used to construct the composite HKB synthesis was used. The citation patterns and the bibliographies of the HKB synthesis were analyzed to see if there could be identified a relatively small set of journals that published what could be assumed to be the most relevant, important, high-quality literature on viral hepatitis. Table VII shows the results of the citation analysis for those articles of the most recent 5-year period referenced in the initial HKB text. It was found that a few journals accounted for a disproportionately large share of the articles cited, yielding a Bradford-like distribution. ('Bradford's law' holds that important information on a topic is contained in a limited number of sources, and that an arithmetic increase in useful information requires a geometric increase in the number of journal article sources [3].) Of the 78 journals contributing articles, 5 journals accounted for nearly 50 % of the citations, 15 journals for nearly 75 %, and only 18 journals accounted for approximately 80 % of the articles cited in the data base synthesis text during this period.

It was hypothesized that if the collaborating experts read all the viral hepatitis articles published by the top 18 journals, the new and important information published on the subject, or references to that information would be obtained. By limitation to a core set of 18 journals for updating, the experts were required to read only 674 articles (67 for each of 10 experts) rather than 5,700 – a much more manageable task.

Data on the initial 2.5-year update plus two subsequent annual updates are shown in table VIII. Of the 1,049 articles randomly distributed to the expert panel, 288 (28 %) were cited at least once; three of the 18 core journals produced no referenced articles. The experts were also encouraged to reference articles published by other journals; they did so, and 20 non-core journals contributed 31 cited articles. Cumulatively, as few as 5 journals accounted for more than 60 % of the citations, and 15 journals accounted for 90 %. Only 10 % of the articles used in the three updating rounds were published by non-core journals. It was concluded that his method of quality filtration of the viral hepatitis literature allows for an effective and efficient means for updating the Hepatitis Knowledge Base contents.

Peptic Ulcer Literature. Following the above studies of the HKB a bibliometric analysis was performed on the bibliographies and citation patterns of the 14 textbook chapters [24] used to create an initial draft Peptic Ulcer Knowledge Base. The 253 pages of gastrointestinal disease text in these chapters contained 2,107 citations to 1,430 enumerated references comprising 1,301 unique documents. The 216 periodical sources cited range in year of publication from 1885 to 1978 with 39 % of their references (540) to literature published in the 6 years prior to the text's 1978 publication

Table VIII. Distribution by journal of 1975 to 1977, 1978, and 1979 articles referenced in update of Hepatitis Knowledge Base

Journal	Number articles distributed for review	Articles referenced by reviewers		cumulative percentage of all referenced
		number	percent	
Lancet	245	62	25	19
Gastroenterology	117	41	35	32
J. infect. Dis.	83	37	46	44
New Engl. J. Med.	133	35	26	55
J. Am. med. Ass	81	22	27	62
Br. med. J.	113	19	33	68
J. Immun.	32	17	53	73
Ann. intern. Med.	49	15	31	78
Am. J. Epidem.	36	12	33	82
Vox Sang.	56	9	16	84
Scand. J. infect. Dis.	21	5	24	86
J. Virol.	14	4	29	87
Proc. Soc. exp. Biol. Med.	15	4	27	88
Nature, Lond.	15	3	20	89
Archs intern. Med.	20	3	15	90
Morbid Mortal Weekly Rep.	0	3	–	91
3 (of 18) journals	19	0	0	91
19 other journals	0	28	–	100
Totals	1,049	319	28	

date (table IX). (Citations to non-periodical literature numbered 110 and accounted for 50 references to 46 distinct documents.)

The bibliographic analysis yielded a journal distribution (see table IX) very reminiscent of that found for viral hepatitis. More than 10 unique articles in each of a group of 21 journals were referenced, accounting for 76% (1,054) of all periodical references; their titles are listed in table IX, column A. The most frequently referenced journal was *Gastroenterology* which accounted for 19% (257) of the total 1,380. Literature published in the most recent 6 years (1972–1978) reveals a similar pattern (see table IX, column E). Of 83 journals and over 540 articles cited during the most recent 6-year period, 1 journal accounted for 21% of the citations; 5 journals accounted

Table IX. Journal sources from text bibliography in peptic ulcer disease most productive of periodical references

1885–1978			1972–1978		
Title A	freq. B	cum. % C	title D	freq. E	cum. % F
1 Gastroenterology	257	19	Gastroenterology	110	21
2 Lancet	97		Lancet	31	
3 Gut	92		Gut	36	
4 Br. med. J.	69		Br. med. J.	28	
5 New Engl. J. Med.	67		New Engl. J. Med.	42	48
6 Am. J. dig. Dis.	66		Am. J. dig. Dis.	18	
7 Am. J. Surg.	50	51	Am. J. Surg.	22	
8 Ann. Surg.	48		Ann. Surg.	23	
9 Gastrointest. Endosc.	40		Gastrointest. Endosc.	37	
10 Scand. J. Gastroent.	38		Scand. J. Gastroent.	24	
11 Archs Surg.	36		Archs Surg.	9	
12 Surgery Gynec. Obstet.	35		Surgery Gynec. Obstet	6	
13 Br. J. Surg.	34		Br. J. Surg.	17	
14 Surgery, St Louis	23		Surgery, St Louis	10	
15 J. Am. med. Ass.	22		J. Am. med. Ass.	8	
16 Q. Jl Med.	15		Ann. intern. Med.	7	
17 Archs intern. Med.	14		J. clin. Invest.	11	75
18 Ann. intern. Med.	14		Radiology	8	
19 J. clin. Invest.	13		Am. J. Gastroent., N.Y.	4	
20 Radiology	13		Aust. N.Z. med. J.	4	
21 Am. J. Roentg.	11	76	Clin. Res.	3	85
	1,054			458	
+60 other multiply cited journals	193	90	+20 other multiply cited journals	40	92
+133 other journals cited once	133		+42 other journals cited once	42	
Totals	1,380	100	Totals	540	100

Table X. Periodical references for MEDLARS files retrieved by a search for literature indexed primarily by peptic ulcer terms

File	Time span	File size	Search postings	Search postings per month	Search Postings as percent of file Size
MEDLINE	1/77–9/79	595,337	2,096 (49% Engl.)	66	0.35
Back 75	1/75–12/76	642,953	2,366 (44% Engl.)	99	0.37
Back 72	1/72–12/74	669,109	2,654 (40% Engl.)	74	0.40
Back 69	1/69–12/71	668,258	2,950 (32% Engl.)	82	0.44
Back 66	1/66–12/68	501,802	2,309 (41% Engl.)	64	0.46

for nearly 48%; 12 journals accounted for 75% and 21 journals accounted for 85% of the articles cited.

A search of MEDLARS bibliographic files (MEDLINE and backfiles) for references to periodical literature primarily indexed under Medical Subject Heading (MeSH) vocabulary terms 'peptic ulcer', 'stomach ulcer', 'duodenal ulcer', 'gastroduodenal ulcer' or 'anti-ulcer agents' was conducted. The postings resulting from this search are summarized in table X. The table shows the total number of documents indexed in each file. The dates shown for the files are dates of accession into the system rather than date of publication, since there is generally a 1- to 2-month lag between receipt of publications and their entry into the data base. Some foreign journals may lag considerably from date of publication to entry due to difficulties in acquisition or translation. There were no significant changes in indexing policy, vocabulary, or journal composition of the MEDLARS data base during this period which might have affected a search for peptic ulcer literature. Two new terms were introduced (Curling's ulcer in 1975 and marginal ulcer in 1964) but both were subsumed under preexisting MeSH terms so the search strategy was unaffected.

From 1969 to the present, an increasing proportion of the peptic ulcer literature cited in the MEDLARS data base has been published in English. Over this period the total number of references primarily indexed under the peptic ulcer search terms used has been steadily decreasing as has been the proportion of the total data base indexed under these terms. A tabulation of the articles found in the MEDLARS files by the ulcer search strategy used for the 21 most productive journals identified from the Sleisenger and Fordtran text bibliography was performed for the 6 years

Table XI. Primary postings of the peptic ulcer literture in a MEDLINE search of 21 selected journals

All MEDLINE files	(1966–1979)	Recent MEDLINE files	(1972–1977)
Gastroenterology	269	Gastroenterology	150
Gut	222	Scand. J. Gastroent.	126
Br. med. J.	216	Gut	106
Br. J. Surg.	189	Br. J. Surg.	96
Lancet	176	Lancet	91
Am. J. Surg.	157	Am. J. dig. Dis.	78
Am. J. dig. Dis.	138	Am. J. Surg.	63
Archs Surg.	120	Ann. Surg.	51
Ann. Surg.	103	Archs. Surg.	46
Surgery, St Louis	79	Surgery, St Louis	34
Surgery Gynec. Obstet.	59	New Engl. J. Med.	29
New Engl. J. Med.	57	Surgery Gynec. Obstet.	24
J. Am. med. Ass.	48	J. Am. med. Ass.	20
Gastrointest. Endosc.	42	Radiology	18
Radiology	31	Gastrointest. Endosc.	13
Q. Jl Med.	8	Ann. intern. Med.	8
Archs intern. Med.	7	J. clin. Invest.	5
J. clin. Invest.	6	Q. Jl Med.	5
Am. J. Roentg.	2	Am. J. Roentg.	1
	2,152[1]		1,065[2]

[1] 2,152 is 43% of 5,035 English postings, and 17.4% of 12,375 total postings.
[2] 1,065 is 37% of 2,868 English postings, and 15.6% of 6,829 total postings.

immediately prior to the textbook publication (1972–1977) (see table XI). The journal sources are ranked by the number of citations elicited by the search strategy. The ranking of these sources is remarkably similar to the ranking from the textbook bibliography, and they account for a significant portion of the total relevant literature. This group of 21 journals accounts in the recent 6-year period for 37% of the English language literature indexed, which is responsive to the primary peptic ulcer query; and for 16% of the total literature (English plus foreign), thus following the Bradford law that there is a concentration of desired information in a small cluster of journals.

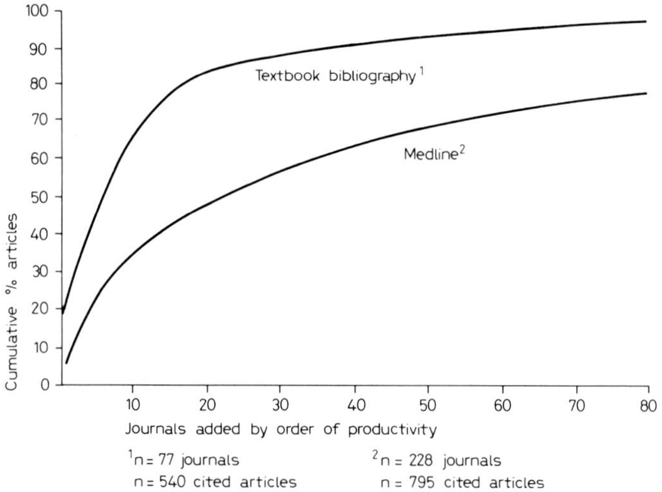

Fig. 7. Distribution of articles on peptic ulcer in journals in Textbook Bibliography and in MEDLINE.

The Bradford distribution of journal sources of relevant citations is shown in figure 7. The upper curve shows the distribution of the contribution of journals to the textbook chapter citations (see data in table IX, column E). The lower similar curve obtains for a MEDLINE search covering literature (795 citations) retrieved by the peptic ulcer search strategy for the period 1978–1980 (see table XII). The comparison indicates that the text bibliography is skewed toward a smaller set of journals containing a large proportion of the important and relevant literature.

It is of interest to compare the references used in the textbook chapters with those obtained from the MEDLINE search for the 21 most productive journals identified from the text bibliography for a 10-year span (1966–1976). The set of postings derived by both methods can be used as a reference standard of 'relevant documents'; this set can be compared to the total retrieval by either system to establish a 'relative retrieval ratio' as a measure of system performance [12]. Table XIII lists the percentages of common postings to those found in the text bibliography and in MEDLINE. Thus, the common postings constituted 40% of the 588 references used in the text chapters, and 14% of the 1,704 references elicited by the MEDLINE search.

From the above data, it is evident that either a MEDLINE search or quality filtered text chapters provide relevant citations to the peptic ulcer

Table XII. Journal ranking of 1978–1980 peptic ulcer articles in MEDLINE

Journal (n = 28)	Articles (number)	Cumulative (percent)
Gastroenterology	48	6
Lancet	45	
Scand. J. Gastroent.	44	
Br. med. J.	39	
Gut	24	
Br. J. Surg.	23	
Am. J. Surg.	20	
Surgery gynec. Ostet.	14	
Sth. med. J.	13	
Wld J. Surg.	13	
Archs Surg.	12	
Aust. N.Z. Surg.	12	
Ann. Surg.	11	
Digestion	10	
Gastroenterol. jap	10	
Med. J. Aust.	10	
New Engl. J. Med.	10	
Surgery, St Louis	10	
Acta chir. scand.	9	
Am. J. dig. Dis.	9	
Dig. Dis. Sci.	9	50
Can. J. Surg.	8	
Gastrointest. Endosc.	8	
Acta gastroenterolg. belg	7	
Acta hepatogastroent.	7	51
+55 other multiply cited journals	198	75
+182 other journals cited once	182	
Total	795	100

Table XIII. Comparison of postings from text bibliography and MEDLINE for peptic ulcer literature in 21 journals (1966–1976) expressed as relative retrieval ratio and percentage

	Ratio of common postings to text postings A	Relative retrieval ratio % B	Ratio of common postings to MEDLINE postings C	Relative retrieval ratio % D
Am. J. dig. Dis.	14/32	44	14/114	12
Am. J. Roentg.	0/8	0	0/0	0
Am. J. Surg.	17/39	44	17/138	12
Ann. intern. Med.	0/7	0	0/5	0
Ann. Surg.	12/76	46	12/84	14
Archs Surg.	13/23	57	13/109	12
Archs intern. Med.	0/5	0	0/5	0
Br. J. Surg.	16/29	55	16/160	10
Br. med. J.	7/130	23	7/159	4
Gastroenterology	51/118	43	51/192	27
Gastrointest. Endosc.	3/42	7	3/36	8
Gut	24/51	47	24/187	13
J. clin. Invest.	5/7	71	5/5	100
J. Am. med. Ass.	1/10	10	1/41	2
Lancet	16/45	36	16/118	14
New Engl. J. Med.	17/41	41	17/44	39
Q. Jl Med.	4/8	50	4/8	50
Radiology	3/9	33	3/22	14
Scand. J. Gastroent.	18/32	56	18/164	11
Surgery Gynec. Obstet.	7/10	70	7/44	16
Surgery, St Louis	10/16	63	10/69	14
Totals	238/588	40	238/1,704	14

literature, but that they give different numbers and arrays of references. Part of the difference can be explained. The MEDLINE search is derived from a comprehensive bibliographic file with no effort made to eliminate redundant or lesser quality information, or to highlight superior quality information. Thus, every 'peptic ulcer' article published by a covered journal will be indexed. Textbook authors seek to document facts and conclusions important to an understanding of the subject, but not necessarily focused entirely on the subject. For example, a textbook author may document the technique of performing an endoscopic procedure in some detail, but the articles cited may not be indexed primarily as 'peptic ulcer' by MEDLINE, and therefore would not be retrieved by the search formulation although present in the data base. Additionally, for economic use of space only selected important subsets of references are cited by authors.

Summary

Bibliometric analyses of the viral hepatitis and peptic ulcer literatures lead to results that are generic in nature, and can be expected to hold for other areas of gastroenterology. They would be useful in construction of knowledge syntheses in additional content areas. There is no need necessarily for gastroenterologists to participate in such bibliometric studies in their fields of interest, but a general understanding of the construction, organization, and distribution of the scientific literature will provide a perspective that will be helpfull in guiding the searcher through the immense and intricate maze toward the specific information needed. Further, bibliometric analyses may be an aid in selection of journals for large institutional or smaller personal libraries.

Conclusion

Gastroenterologists face the same information retrieval problems as in other fields of biomedicine and indeed all of science and technology. Whatever processes are used, the best decisions require use of the current state of knowledge. 'Current knowledge' is spread throughout an immense and complicated literature. The primary journal literature is immense. The synthesized tertiary literature is immense. The secondary literature – indexing and abstracting – has grown in size and has generated remarkable new aids for finding needed information. Extravagantly large numbers and techniques of publications are used to facilitate linking of the individual user with the information needed. Advances in computer and communications technology have made bibliographic approaches orders of magnitude more effective and efficient over the past two decades. New extensions of these technologies can now be seen moving into support and delivery of both primary and tertiary literature, and can be expected to revolutionize the delivery of medical information over the next decade.

In the face of all this, what should the gastroenterologist do? When all is said and done, information retrieval is an individual problem. The individual user must define what it is that is needed. Defining that individual information need is the most crucial single step toward satisfying it, for, as described in this chapter, there is a vast and changing information network out there trying, in ever so many ways, to link the world's available knowledge to the user's information needs. The more one understands what is out there, the more likely that linkage can occur. Finally, information specialists and medical librarians can be of enormous help as intermediaries between the searcher and the systems.

References

1 Ackoff, R.L.; Designing a national scientific and technical communication system (University of Pennsylvania Press, Philadelphia 1976).

2 Bernstein, L.M.; Siegel, E.R.; Goldstein, C.M.: The hepatitis knowledge base: a prototype information transfer system. Ann. intern. Med. *93*: 169–181 (1980).

3 Bradford, S.C.: Documentation, pp. 144–159 (Crosby, Lockwood & Son, London 1953).

4 Branscomb, L.M.: The misinformation explosion: is the literature worth reviewing? Sci. Res. *3*: 49–56 (1968).

5 Cummings, M.M.: The National Library of Medicine and quality information filters; in Warren, Goffman, Coping with the biomedical literature explosion: a qualitative approach. Working papers, pp. 61–67 (Rockefeller Foundation, New York 1978).

6 Etzioni, A.: The need for quality filters in information systems (Editorial). Science *171*: 133 (1971).

7 Garfield, E.: Citation analysis as a tool in journal evaluation. Science *178*: 471–479 (1972).

8 Herring, C.: Distill or drown; the need for reviews. Physics Today *21*: 27–33 (1968).

9 Hiltz, S.R.; Turoff, M.: The network nation (Addison-Wesley Publishing, Reading 1978).

10 Huth, E.J.: An information system for the future (editorial). Ann. intern. Med. *93*: 139–140 (1980).

11 King, D.W.; McDonald, D.D.; Roderer, N.K.; Wood, B.L.: Statistical indicators of scientific and technical communication (1960–1980). vol. I (King Research, Rockville 1976).

12 Lancaster, F.W.: Information retrieval systems: characteristics, testing and evaluation (Wiley, New York 1979).

13 Lister Hill National Center for Biomedical Communications, National Library of Medicine. The hepatitis knowledge base (short form). Ann. intern. Med. *93*: 183–222 (1980).

14 McCarn, D.B.: National Library of Medicine – MEDLARS and MEDLINE; in Belzer, Holzman, Kent, Encyclopedia of computer science and technology, vol. II, pp. 116–152 (Dekker, New York 1978).

15 Mosley, J.W.; Galambos, J.T.: Viral Hepatitis; in Schiff, Diseases of the liver; 4th edition, pp. 500–593 (Lippincott, Philadelphia 1975).

16 Pao, M.L.: A quality filtering system for medical literature. J. med. Educ. *50*: 353–359 (1975).

17 Proceedings of a symposium on viral hepatitis. National Academy of Sciences, vol. I. Am. J. med. Sci. *270*: 2–209 (1975).

18 Proceedings of a symposium on viral hepatitis. National Academy of Sciences, vol. II. Am. J. med. Sci. *270*: 213–412 (1975).

19 Roderer, N.K.: US Expenditures for biomedical communication: 1960–1985 (King Research, Rockville 1979).

20 Roderer, N.K.; King, D.W.; McDonald, D.D.; Bush, D.G.: Evaluation of the hepatitis knowledge base (King Research, Rockville 1981).

21 Siegel, E.R.: Use of computer conferencing to validate and update NLMs hepatitis knowledge base; in Henderson, MacNaughton, The future of electronic communications (Am. Association for the Advancement of Science, Washington 1980).

22 Siegel, E.R.: Transfer of information to health practitioners; in Dervin, Voight, Progress in communication sciences, vol. III, pp. 311–334 (Ablex Publishing, Norwood 1982).

23 Siegel, E.R.; Sneiderman, C.A.; Falkenberg, G.C.W.; Fraser, G.R.: Quality filtration of the published biomedical literature: some methods and strategies; in Cosmides, Proc. Symp. on Information Transfer in Toxicology, pp. 99–109 (National Library of Medicine, Bethesda 1981).

24 Sleisenger, M.H.; Fordtran, J.S.: Gastrointestinal disease; 2nd ed. (Saunders, Philadelphia 1978).

25 Touloukian, Y.S.: The end of science for evaluated information. Bull. Am. Soc. Information Sci. 5: 44 (1979).

26 Urquart, D.S.: The use of scientific periodicals; in Int. Conf. on Scientific Information, pp. 277–290 (National Academy of Sciences, Washington 1958).

27 Warren, K.S.; Goffman, W.: Analysis of a medical literature: a case study; in Warren, Goffman, Coping with the biomedical literature explosion: a qualitative approach. Working papers, pp. 31–53 (Rockefeller Foundation, New York 1978).

28 Ziman, J.M.: Public knowledge (Cambridge University Press, Cambridge 1968).

L.M. Bernstein, MD, Department of Health and Human Services,
National Institutes of Health, National Library of Medicine, Building 38A,
Room 7S718, Bethesda, MD 20209 (USA)

Front. gastrointest. Res., vol. 7, pp. 186–191 (Karger, Basel 1984)

Future Progress for Computer Aids in Gastro-Enterology

F.T. de Dombal

Clinical Information Science Group, University of Leeds, Leeds, England

Previous chapters in this volume have set out in some detail a series of possible roles for computer assistance in gastro-enterological practice. In each chapter the author concerned has described the current state of the art in the relevant field – sometimes referring to specific projects and problems, sometimes presenting a more general overview of the situation.

In this final chapter we shall attempt to look beyond the current situation and discuss the possible future for computer assistance in clinical gastro-enterological practice. In particular the discussion in this final chapter will focus on a number of crucial factors on which future progress would seem to depend.

Factor 1: The Effectiveness of Current Programs

As discussed elsewhere in this volume, there is a quaint notion amongst computer people that physicians are old-fashioned, reactionary creatures – almost pathologically antagonistic to the concepts of high technology. This is demonstrable nonsense; since the age of the stethoscope was ushered in by *Laennec*, it has been virtually impossible to keep physicians away from high technology. Indeed, one of the biggest problems of the present era is to *stop* physicians using high technology where low technology (or no technology at all) will solve their problem!

We therefore reject utterly the concept that 'Luddite' physicians dismiss computer systems out of hand. All too often physicians dismiss computer programs and systems which are demonstrated to them *because they do not fulfil the needs of the physicians concerned*. Either the systems don't work, or they don't do what the physician wants, or they do what the physician wants but at enormous cost in terms of material or effort, or they are unreliable, or they are over-sold by enthusiastic champions of computers, or some combination of these factors.

Future progress for computer assistance in clinical gastro-enterological practice will depend, above anything else, upon development in the next few years of simple practical programs which meet the needs of the physicians concerned. If this is not done, then the medical profession will reject the computer aid, and in these circumstances it would be perfectly right and proper for them so to do.

Factor 2: Hardware Developments

To take a somewhat more hopeful view – given that in the next few years systems *do* emerge which meet the perceived needs of clinicians in gastro-enterology (and at acceptable cost) – one may then ask a series of supplementary questions about other factors in computing practice which might affect further development and improvement in these computer aids.

The computer field is a fast-moving one, and nowhere more so than in hardware development. It becomes relevant therefore to ask what developments in computer (hardware) technology might appear in the foreseeable future which would effect clinician's acceptance and use of such systems. Actually, although a number of developments can obviously be anticipated, many of these would seem only distantly related to routine use in gastro-enterological practice. Nevertheless, there are some developments on the horizon which merit discussion; and undoubtedly the two developments which *should* effect the situation are: (1) increasing computer storage capacity, and (2) increasing ease of communication between clinician and computer.

As regards the former, computer storage is increasing almost exponentially, and it seems reasonable to suppose that – well within 2 years – microsystems with 256KB of central storage and megabytes of disc storage will be readily accessible in most gastro-enterological departments, at a price approximating to that of current microcomputers or personal computers. This will enable the doctor to store any data he wishes (within reason) about his patient population, the constraint on such storage being the ability of humans to enter the data rather than the computer to hold and retrieve it.

Equally important with increasing storage are developments in prospect which will influence progress in clinical practice by influencing the ease with which doctors can communicate with their computer. At the moment such developments as light pens, touch-sensitive screens and systems which have the ability to read hand-writing (particularly clinicians' hand-writing!) are either relatively untested or expensive. It can be anticipated, however, that in the coming 3–5 years these aids to clinicians' input of data into the computer will become more widespread, and more attractively priced. Since a number of previous studies have shown that doctors are currently ineffective and relatively reluctant computer users, undoubtedly this type of improvement will effect future progress to a considerable degree.

Factor 3: Improvements in Software Packages

We have already commented upon the current importance of the *effectiveness* of computer programs which are offered to physicians. It goes without saying that the future progress in gastro-enterology of computer aids will be critically dependent upon the development of software packages which meet the objectives and perceived needs of clinicians. In these paragraphs we briefly consider some additional aspects of software package developments.

First, software packages can now be written in languages which are intelligible to clinicians – at least to a significant minority of them. Future software package developers will need to consider very carefully both the advantages and disadvantages of writing programs which the user can understand. (There is no clear-cut answer to this problem, and the matter is mentioned as a basic for debate.) Should future software packages be readily intelligible to the majority of users so that they can 'see what is going off' inside the computer? Or, on the other hand, is it desirable that physicians should be *deliberately prevented* from access to this type of knowledge, possibly on the grounds that it would be confusing for them and possibly dangerous by causing them to make assumptions which are not in fact warranted. (An excellent example of this problem concerns the current debate over the use of the Bayes theorem, see p. 122.) Indeed, exactly the same questions will need to be raised and answered as were presented to society in the middle-ages by the development of printing presses.

One further factor upon which future progress will depend concerns *net-working*. Essentially two questions need to be answered. First, what should be net-worked? Should *whole systems* be net-worked which consist of a computer and program (possibly hardwired into it in a special EPROM chip)? Or should *software packages* be developed which are virtually machine-independent, so that what one is distributing is simply a program? Or should one distribute *concepts* and leave local research personnel to work out an individual solution by means of a program tailored to that specific locality?

To some extent the answer depends upon a further question. If programs are to be developed which have application in more than one locality, to what extent can variation in clinical practice by geographical locality be predicted and overcome? Essentially the program here hinges upon the degree to which doctors in different localities can be induced to adopt a common or unified terminology. This problem is addressed elsewhere by Dr. *Jeanty* (p. 46) and whether the particular solution proposed by Dr. *Jeanty* (SNOMED) is right or wrong undoubtedly something along these lines will be necessary before 'general' systems can be developed for use in more than one location.

Finally, the effectiveness and attractiveness of software packages will undoubtedly be enhanced by the development in 'aids to presentation'. To study this point one has merely to look at the development of computer games; since crucial in their development were those improvements in software packaging which allowed such games to be presented more realistically and (visually) more attractively. The so-called 'space invaders' derivatives are an excellent example of an explosion in computer use following improvements in presentation. Undoubtedly we may look to similar developments in packages for gastro-enterologists, particularly in terms of 'house-keeping' programs diagnostic programs and teaching programs.

Factor 4: Resource Allocation

A further factor which will clearly govern future progress is the extent to which resources are allocated to the development of computer aids in gastro-enterology. This is at first sight a somewhat worrying problem, since resource allocation is becoming ever more restricted nowadays – in the light of present world circumstances. Even though much computer aid is instituted in the name of 'rationalisation' and 'saving resources', it would be unrealistic to except vast expansion of resources devoted to the development of these aids in the immediate future.

Ideally one would like to see the development of computer aids proceed on the 'ladder' principle. That is to say two types of effort take place at the same time. The first arm is '*basic research*', designed to develop further packages in the future and improve upon existing ones. The second arm of this development is '*operational*', in which existing packages are implemented under carefully controlled conditions and their use rigorously monitored in a defined clinical situation. In this way additional information is secured which can then be 'fed back' to those developing new packages and improving existing ones. The two 'arms' of this project are therefore totally interdependent.

There is thus a role for quite a wide variety of grant funding agencies in terms of provision of research. Perhaps this role may be more clearly defined as follows: (a) some grant funding bodies (such as Research Councils) may need to be more closely involved with the *basic medical research* necessary to construct packages in the first place; (b) local sources (such as local hospital funds) will need to be involved in the provision of resources so that packages which have been developed can be *clinically implemented*, and (c) there is clearly a role for national and possibly supra-national agencies (such as government departments, the European Community or even WHO) in the *careful monitoring* of existing packages so as to evaluate their use as rigorously as possible and to promulgate (as widely as possible) existing successful packages.

It is arguable that in recent years these three areas of resource provision have not been well integrated, and in particular (in many countries) the relationships between those testing developed systems and those involved in basic studies have been poor. This has acted to supress existing systems and hinder their development. Perhaps therefore it is the *co-ordination* of resource allocation, rather than its magnitude, which will determine future progress.

Factor 5: Physicians' Reactions

Undoubtedly, however, the most important factor in the development of computer aids to gastro-enterology will be the reaction towards these systems of physicians. From time to time computer-orientated articles appear in the literature, forecasting the demise of the doctor and the replacement of 'mere' clinicians by more rational systems! It has to be said that this sort of nonsense is totally unrealistic; and in the foreseeable future the pivot upon which gastro-enterological practice will hinge will be the gastro-enterologist. This would be held to be self evident by some.

However, an important corollary of this concerns gastro-enterological computer aids: for, if the pivot of the system is the physician, then whatever systems are developed must: (a) meet the perceived needs of the physician, and (b) be constructed in such a way as to appear reasonably attractive to the user. The phrase 'user-friedly' is familiar and trite. One current advertising slogan (for a computer called a DRAGON) claims that it is so 'user-friendly' that it practically licks your hand! But nowhere is this more important than in the interaction between computer systems and practising clinicians. Computer systems which (in this sense) lick physicians' hands are vital.

Of course, in the future this will change. The average young doctor in the 1990s will (in developed countries at any rate) have been brought up in an educational system where routine usage of computers is the rule rather than the exception. Such a doctor might be expected to have grown up in a home environment which includes a computer system and may well be thoroughly familiar with the type of computer system outlined in the preceding pages even before arrival in medical school.

However, in the immediate future (i.e. the next 10 years) such computer literacy cannot be taken for granted and it will be the end of the century before this type of 'computer-literate' doctor arrives in a position of sufficient seniority to influence progress significantly. In the meantime, it is mandatory that awareness of gastro-enterologists about computers, their strengths and inherent problems, their role in gastro-enterological practice, and (above all) their limitations, should be enhanced by whatever means are available.

Undoubtedly the best method of achieving this is with the use of computers themselves. Nothing instructs like 'hand-on' experience. Nevertheless, such experience will not be possible in the immediate future on anything other than a limited scale; and there is thus clearly a place for a more leisurely approach – in which the gastro-enterologist can thoughtfully consider: (a) what computer aids are available, and (b) how they might help his clinical practice. To assist this process has been the aim of the present volume.

F.T. de Dombal, MD, Reader in Clinical Information Science, Room 8, Level 5, Clinical Sciences Building, St. James Hospital, Leeds LS9 7TF (England)

Subject Index